Sports Analytics in Practice with R

Sports Analytics in Practice with R

Ted Kwartler
Harvard Extension School
Adjunct, Faculty of Arts & Sciences
Maynard, MA

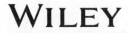

Registered Offices
John Wiley & Sons, Inc., 111 River Street, Hoboken, NJ 07030, USA
John Wiley & Sons Ltd, The Atrium, Southern Gate, Chichester, West Sussex, PO19 8SQ, UK

Editorial Office
9600 Garsington Road, Oxford, OX4 2DQ, UK

For details of our global editorial offices, customer services, and more information about Wiley products visit us at www.wiley.com.

Wiley also publishes its books in a variety of electronic formats and by print-on-demand. Some content that appears in standard print versions of this book may not be available in other formats.

Library of Congress Cataloging-in-Publication Data
Names: Kwartler, Ted, 1978- author.
Title: Sports analytics in practice with R / Ted Kwartler, Maynard, MA.
Description: First Edition. | Hoboken, NJ : John Wiley & Sons, Inc., 2022. | Includes bibliographical
    references and index. | Contents: Introduction to R -- Data Vizualization & Dashboards: Best practices --
    Geospatial Data: Understanding changing baseball player behavior -- Machine Learning Basics: Modeling
    football draft patterns, pick number & clusters among athletes -- Logistic Regression: Explaining basketball
    wins & losses with coefficients -- Natual Language Processing: Understanding cricket fan topics & sentiment --
    Linear Optimization: Programmatically seleting an optimal fantasy football lineup.
Identifiers: LCCN 2021042430 (print) | LCCN 2021042431 (ebook) | ISBN 9781119598077 (Hardback) |
    ISBN 9781119598060 (PDF) | ISBN 9781119598091 (ePub) | ISBN 9781119598084 (eBook)
Subjects: LCSH: Sports--Statistics. | Mathematical statistics--Computer programs. |
    R (Computer program language)
Classification: LCC GV706.8 .K85 2022 (print) | LCC GV706.8 (ebook) | DDC 796.02/1--dc23/eng/20211020
LC record available at https://lccn.loc.gov/2021042430
LC ebook record available at https://lccn.loc.gov/2021042431

Cover image: © Lorado/Getty Images
Cover design by Wiley

Set in 9.5/12.5pt STIXTwoText by Integra Software Services Pvt. Ltd, Pondicherry, India

C9781119598077_240222

Printed and bound by CPI Group (UK) Ltd, Croydon CR0 4YY

Contents

Preface

Sports is one of the few places where the data and outcomes are well known. Unlike medicine which requires significant subject-matter expertise or business where the data is proprietary in most cases, sports knowledge is relatively accessible, and the data and outcomes are public. As a result, sports analytics serves as a great entry point for many aspiring data scientists and analytics professionals. For the novice, this book demonstrates the many facets and uses of countless techniques applicable outside of sports. It should have more than enough topics and examples to aid learning for general practice. For the avid R programmer and sports fan, the book likely has some new functions and techniques which may be less well known. These readers will delight in improving and expanding the demonstrated methods once the core concepts are understood. Finally, for those already in the sports analytics world the techniques and individual chapter topics can serve as a reference and starting point in their professional analysis. For instance, much of the use cases in the chapters can be adjusted to specific sports or updated by more recent underlying data.

This book has been a long journey in the making. Originally the book's scope was centered on individualized chapters demonstrating analytical techniques within a sports context. The goal is that a reader inherits various tools that act as a foundation for analysis to build upon and add complexity with subsequent analyses as the reader's technical acumen and sports interests grow. Each chapter is meant to be a standalone reference as the reader explores and learns. This also frees up the reader to focus on topics of interest. For example, a reader may not want to learn about natural language processing so could skip that chapter altogether to focus on another subject such as optimizing a fantasy football lineup. The book's undertaking grew in complexity due to a personal commitment to demonstrate concepts on diverse data sets including Paralympic athletes, female soccer and basketball, and less US-centric popular sports including cricket in addition to the more typically demonstrated sports analyses of men's football, baseball, and basketball. My goal is to make the subject accessible and relevant to many in the analytics field despite this effort slowing the book's creation. Keep in mind a chapter's concepts can be applied to many sports domains. For example, the text analysis applied to cricket fan forum posts can easily be applied to men's basketball fan tweets or forum posts. Each chapter's takeaway is meant to be a broadly useful tool, not a brittle or narrowly focused analysis. Additionally, the book was delayed due to the pandemic's effect on the sports-world. Admittedly the shortened seasons, canceled games, and other changes that created outlier statistics pales in comparison to the pandemic's hardship and humanistic impact outside of sports. Despite these challenges, the book's end result was worth the delay. The final product covers many diverse concepts, and data, encouraging analytics professionals to enjoy the intersection of sports and analysis.

The book's supporting website is www.rstatsbook.com. The site contains data and scripts along with any code revisions necessary as functions and packages change. Redundantly, data is shared via git repository at www.github.com/kwartler/Practical_Sports_Analytics.

Author Biography

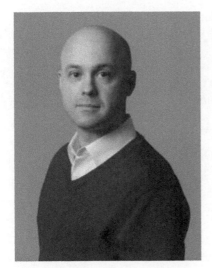

Ted Kwartler
Adjunct Professor, Harvard University

Ted Kwartler is the VP, Trusted AI at DataRobot. At DataRobot, Ted sets product strategy for explainable and ethical uses of data technology in the company's application. Ted brings unique insights and experience utilizing data, business acumen, and ethics to his current and previous positions at Liberty Mutual Insurance and Amazon. In addition to having four DataCamp courses, he teaches graduate courses at the Harvard Extension School and is the author of Text Mining in Practice with R.

Analytics don't work at all. It's just some crap some people who were really smart made up.

Charles Barkley, former NBA player

Just because you don't understand something doesn't mean it's crap.

Ross Drucker, NBA Future Analytics Stats Program Analyst

My dear Nora & Brenna,

My inspiration and guides. I wrote this book in your honor though don't expect either of you to follow my footsteps into analysis. Your journey is your own, may you find a passion and, if desirable, have the opportunity to write about it. No matter where your attention and intellect lead you I remain.

Your loving father,
Ted

Foreword

Writing a book is no easy task yet for some reason I decided to write a second! Overall, I am grateful to the countless people that helped me learn, expand, and apply these methods. Data science and analytics is as much as "team sport" as any, where collaboration, communication, and effort often wins the day.

First I would like to acknowledge Jack W, whose intellect and athleticism left us far too early. For anyone struggling with mental health, know that you are loved, you are valuable, and people in your community are here for you. Your passing was a motivating reminder of the short time we have to make contributions along with the need for more kindness toward those that may be suffering silently.

Next, Anup B, one of the most brilliant supportive leaders I have worked for. Not to mention your passion for cricket helped open my eyes to a noteworthy and enjoyable sport. Losing you to the pandemic was a disturbing blow felt by many people who were touched by your intelligence, humor, and positivity.

This entire book would not have been possible without the fine professors at the University of Notre Dame that put me on my own professional journey. I fondly remember building my first logistic regression predicting March Madness after learning these techniques from Dr. Keating, the late Dr. Gilbride, and Dr. Devaraj.

Further I would like to acknowledge my parents, Anatol and Trish, and my endearing wife, Meghan. Your support and patience has been significant. Writing a book is no small undertaking with much of the logistical burden falling to each of you. Completing this book is a shared victory.

Lastly, my sincerest gratitude to the wonderful team at Wiley, particularly Kimberly Monroe-Hill. Your patience and flexibility to late submissions and delayed seasons stemming from the unusual 2020 year in sports (among other more important hardships) has been greatly appreciated. I was ready to give up on the project yet your e-mails demonstrated a commitment from Wiley that I cherish.

1

Introduction to R

Objectives

- Learn about R as a programming language
- Define Integrated Development Environment
- Define objects
- Learn the assignment operator
- Define functions
- Executing a loop
- Learn logical operators
- Learn about R data types
- Learn about object classes
- Indexing data objects
- Extending R functionality with packages
- Writing a custom function
- Create a scatter plot with sports data
- Create a heatmap with sports data

R Libraries

```
ggplot2
ggthemes
RCurl
tidyr
```

R Functions

```
+
plot
<-
round
```

Sports Analytics in Practice with R, First Edition. Ted Kwartler.
© 2022 John Wiley & Sons Ltd. Published 2022 by John Wiley & Sons Ltd.

```
class
as.factor
as.character
c
cbind
rbind
data.frame
as.matrix
as.data.frame
install.packages
library
getURL
read.csv
dim
names
head
tail
summary
table
qplot
pivot_longer
geom_tile
scale_fill_gradient
xlab
ggtitle
theme
theme_hc
```

The R Programming Language

R is an open-source, freely available programming language used throughout this book. R is a powerful and longstanding programming language developed more than 20 years ago. It is a derivative of the "S" programming language for statistics originating in the mid-1990s developed by AT&T and Lucent Technologies. Unlike other programming languages, R is optimized specifically for statistics including but not limited to simulation, machine learning, visualizations, and traditional statistical modeling (linear regression) as well as tests. Due to the open-source nature of R, many developers, academics, and enthusiasts have contributed to its development for their specific needs. As a result, the language is extensible meaning it can be easily used for various purposes. For example, through R markdown, simple websites and presentations can be created. In another use case, R can be used for traditional linear modeling or machine learning and can draw upon various data types for analysis including audio files, digital images, text, numeric, and various other data files and types. Thus, it is widely used and nonspecialized other than to say R is an analysis language. This differs from other languages which specialize in web development like Ruby or python which has extended its functionality to building applications not just analysis.

In this textbook, the R language is applied specifically to sports contexts. Of course, the code in this book can be used to extend your understanding of sports analytics. It may give you insights to a particular sport or analytical aspect within the sport itself such as what statistics should be focused on to win a basketball game. However, learning the code in this book can also help open up a world of analytical capabilities beyond sports. One of the benefits of learning statistics, programming, and various analysis methods with sports data is that the data is widely available and outcomes are known. This means that your analysis, models, and visualizations can be applied, and you can review the outcomes as you expand upon what is covered in this book. This differs from other programming and statistical examples which may resort to boring, synthetic data to illustrate an analytical result. Using sports data is realistic and can be future oriented, making the learning more challenging yet engaging. Modeling the survivors of the Titanic pales in comparison since you cannot change the historical outcome or save future cruise ship mates. Thus, modeling which team will win a match or which player is a good draft pick is a superior learning experience.

If you are new to programming don't be intimidated. R is a forgiving language in that things like spacing an indentation are ignored. Further, the R community is well supported and a simple online search of any error message usually finds an answer quickly on any number of sites.

To begin your R and sports analytics journey, please download the "base-R" distribution for your operating system. The "Comprehensive R Archive Network," CRAN, is the home of the official R distribution as well as officially supported packages (more on that in a bit). The site to download base-R is https://cran.r-project.org.

Unfortunately, base-R, having started in the nineties, looks abysmal and lacks some modern day functionality. Thus, you will need to next download the R-Studio Integrated Development Environment, or IDE. An IDE is software that consolidates many of the aspects needed to code into one place. For example, you will need to write code which could be done in a simple notepad like program, a place to execute the code written, a place to visualize plots that were output from the code, and so on. These individual components are assembled into the IDE for ease of use and fast development. R and many other languages have IDEs. In fact, R has multiple IDE optimized for the type of analysis you are performing such as biostatistics or working with another language like Java. The most popular and easily supported IDE for base-R is the R-Studio software. There are server and desktop versions available. The code executed in this book should work for either cloud or local but installation of base-R and R-Studio on a server is not covered. Therefore, please download the R-Studio *desktop* IDE by navigating to https://www.rstudio.com/products/rstudio.

The R-Studio IDE, or Integrated Development Environment, adds functionality and modern user interface to base-R. The IDE aggregates common functionality used for software development and statistical analysis.

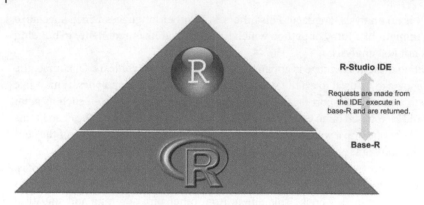

Figure 1.1 The relationship between base-R and R-studio.

Essentially R-Studio sits on top of base-R. The IDE provides a modern GUI expected of today's computer users while also adding functionality including the use of version control, terminal access and perhaps most importantly an easy way to create and view visualizations for easy export and saving to disk. Figure 1.1 illustrates the basic relationship for base-R and R-Studio. As you can see without base-R, the IDE will not function because none of the computational functions exist in the IDE itself.

Now that you have both base-R and R-Studio, let's start to explore the programming environment. Think of an R environment as a relatively generic statistical piece of software. Once downloaded it can perform all tasks programmatically found in many of the popular spread sheet programs either online or for a laptop. The advantage of R is its extensibility mentioned earlier. R can be specialized from a generic statistical set of tools into a more interesting and nuanced piece of software. This is done through the download of specialized packages and called in the console by loading the package for the task at hand.

Figure 1.2 shows the IDE itself without a "script" to be executed. For now, focus on the "console" section in Figure 1.2. This is the lower left-hand side containing a ">" symbol. This is the section where code will be executed and results are returned.

The next step is to navigate to "File > New File > R Script" in the upper left of the IDE. This will open another pane in the IDE. The script pane will be located in the upper left section of the IDE and will shrink the console on the lower left-hand side. While the console is where code is executed and computation enacted, the scripting section is where you will write code that is then run within the console. Think of an R script as merely a lightweight text file that can be saved and repeated by running in the console. A script is nothing more than a set of instructions that have not been enacted yet. To save an R script, navigate to "File > Save" and then simply follow the IDE dialog. The rest of the book provides R scripts for you to execute along with explanations along the way. Figure 1.3 shows the new script pane with some basic example code.

Of particular note in the script shown in Figure 1.3 are two comments and two code examples. A comment begins with a `#`. This tells R to ignore everything on that line. As you begin your learning journey programming in R, it is a best practice to add comments to remind yourself the nuances of the code to be executed. Thus, feel free to make a copy of any scripts throughout the book, add comments, and save for yourself.

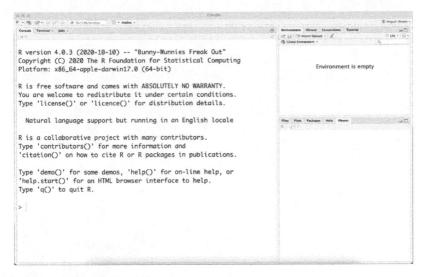

Figure 1.2 The R-Studio IDE console.

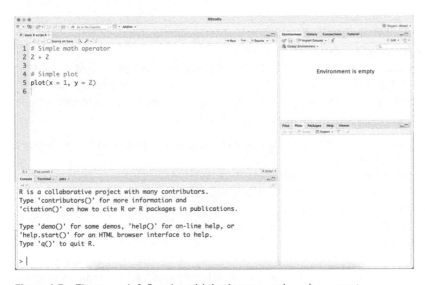

Figure 1.3 The upper left R script with basic commands and comments.

The first code to be executed, beginning on a non-commented line, is a simple arithmetic operation shown below.

```
2 + 2
```

Since this is in a script, it will not be run until you declare it within the console. Further, as you can guess the operation `2 + 2` has a single result `4`. An easy way to run the script is to place your cursor on the line you want to execute and click the "run" icon on the upper right-hand side of the script. When this is done the code is transferred to the

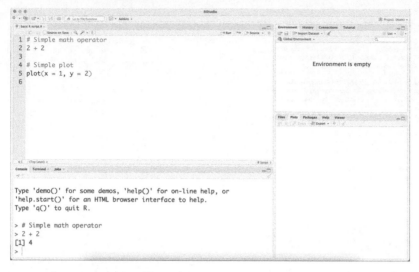

Figure 1.4 Showing the code execution on line 2 of the script being transferred to the console where the result 4 is printed.

console and executed, returning the single answer as expected. Figure 1.4 illustrates the transfer between script and console.

Next, let's execute another command which will illustrate another pane of the IDE. If your cursor is on line 5 of the R script, `plot(x = 1, y = 2)` and you click the "run" icon you will now see a simple scatter plot visual appear in the lower right utility pane titled "Plots." Each tab of the utility pane is described below:

- **Files**—This is a file navigation view, where you can review folders and files to be used in analysis or saved to disk.
- **Plots**—For reviewing any static visualizations the R code creates. This pane can also be used for resizing the image using a graphical user interface (GUI) and saving the plots to disk.
- **Packages**—Since R needs to be specialized for a particular task, this pane lists your local package library with official documentation and accompanying examples, vignettes, and tutorials.
- **Help**—Provides various resources for obtaining help with R and its many tasks.
- **Viewer**—This pane allows you to view the small webpages and dynamic interactive plots which R can create.

Figure 1.5 shows the result of a basic, yet not visually appealing scatter plot with a single point. Rest assured the plots throughout the book are more compelling than this simplistic example. The x,y coordinate points are defined in code as `x = 1` and `y = 2`.

Next, let's focus on the remaining upper right pane of the IDE. The primary tab of interest is the "Environment" tab. R works by creating objects which are stored data objects. When an object is created, it is held in active memory, your computer's RAM. Any active objects in your R session will be shown in the "Environment" tab in the upper right. Add the following code in the script (upper left) pane, then click "run" to instantiate an object in your environment. Notice the first bit follows a `#` so the non-code comment "Create

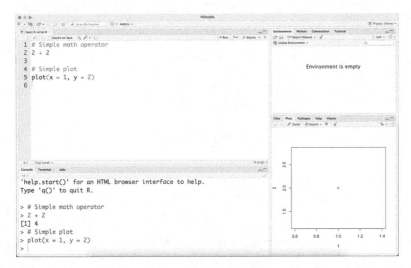

Figure 1.5   The basic scatter plot is instantiated in the lower right, "Plots" plane.

an object" acts as a signpost for you while the next line actually creates the object. Specifically, the object name is `xVal` and it is declared have a value of `1`. Moreover, the declaration of the object name to value is done with the assignment operate `<-`. In the R language you can also use an equal sign for the object name assignment. However, most R style guides use the `<-` operator and this book follows that direction.

```
# Create an object
xVal <- 1
```

When run the upper right environment tab will now show an object, `xVal`, that is held in memory for use later in the script. Of course, these objects can become much more complex than a single value. Next add more code to your script utilizing the `xVal` object rather than declaring the value explicitly. The following code can be added to your script and then run to recreate the simple scatter plot from before. The difference is that R has substituted the `x = xVal` input to `x = 1` since that is the object's actual value. The only difference in the plots is that the second one has a different *x*-axis title because the value was derived from the object name. Figure 1.6 now shows the additional code chunks, the new object in the environment, and the recreated plot in the utility pane.

```
# Create a plot with an object value
plot(x = xVal, y = 2)
```

The basic functionality of R is underpinned by functions and objects. Each package that specializes R comes with a set of functions usually coordinated for a particular task like data manipulation, obtaining sports data or similar. Functions accept inputs, including objects, and manipulate the inputs most often to create new objects or to overwrite and replace existing objects. For example, the following code creates a new object `newObj` using the assignment operator and on the right-hand side employs a base-R function. Base-R functions do not require any libraries to be loaded, so there is no need

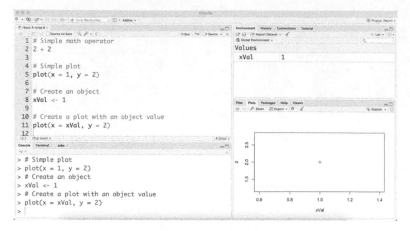

Figure 1.6   The renewed plot with an R object in the environment.

to specialize the R environment for a particular task. The `newObj` variable is declared as a result of a function `round` with two input parameters. The first parameter accepts the number to be rounded, `1.23`. The second parameter `digits = 0` is a tuning parameter which changes the behavior of the `round` function declaring the number of decimals to round the input to. Thus, when you add the following code to the script and then execute it in the console, the resulting `newObj` variable has a corresponding value of 1. As before, the `newObj` object will be stored actively and shown in the "Environment" tab. Keep in mind the inputs themselves can be objects not just declared values. As a result of this behavior, scripts manipulate objects and often pass them to another function later in the script.

```
# Create a new object with a function
newObj <- round(1.23, digits = 0)
```

This book will illustrate many functions both in base-R and within specialized packages applied in a sports context. R has many tens of thousands of packages with corresponding functions. Often the rest of this book will defer to base-R functions in an effort for standardization, stability, and ease of understanding rather than utilize an esoteric package. This is a deliberate choice to improve conceptual understanding but does leave room for code optimization and improvement.

There are additional intermediate programming operators that are employed in this book. In fact, there are multiple types of logical and arithmetic operators but for the most part the scripts in this book are focused on one use case at a time, with linear thinking, so you can focus on the concepts and applications more so than concise code. However, Table 1.1 describes the three control flow operators used in the book with a code example for you to try in your script and console. Within the FOR loop, a set of code is run repeatedly with a variable that changes each time through. For the latter two, the IF and IFELSE control flows, a logical statement is evaluated and controls the code's behavior. If the statement is run and returns TRUE, then the code is executed otherwise it is ignored.

Table 1.1 Three simple control flows in R including the FOR loop, IF and IFELSE statement.

Name	Code	Description
FOR loops	```for (i in 1:4){ print(i + 2) }```	The FOR loop has a dynamic variable `i` which will update a number of times. Here, the `i` value loop will repeat from 1, 2, 3, and 4. The code within the curly brackets executes with the updated `i` value. The first time through the loop `i` equals `1` and with `+ 2` the value 3 is printed to the console. The second time through `i` updates to `2` and is once again added with `+ 2` so that the value `4` is printed. This continues in the loop 4 times because of the `1:4` parameter
IF statement	```if(xVal == 1){ print('xVal is equal to one.') }```	The IF statement is a control operator. After the `if` code, a statement is created to check its validity. If the statement inside parentheses evaluates to TRUE, then the code within the curly brackets is executed. In this example, the statement checks whether a variable `xVal` is equal to `1`. Since it does, the code in the curly brackets executes and a message is printed to the console state "xVal is equal to one." If the statement does not evaluate to TRUE, the code inside the curly brackets is ignored. For example, if `xVal == 2`, then the code block is not run
IF ELSE statement	```if(xVal == 1){ print('xVal is equal to one.') } else { print('xVal is not equal to one.') }```	The IF-ELSE control flow adds another layer to the previous IF statement. Now a new set of curly brackets is added along with the `else` function. This statement will execute one of the two code chunks within the curly brackets based on the TRUE or FALSE result of the logical statement. Here, if `xVal == 1`, then the first message is printed, same as before. However, for any other value of `xVal`, the second bit of code is run. For example, if `xVal == 2`, then the IF statement evaluates to FALSE and the second message "xVal is not equal to one" will be printed to the console.

Another aspect of R programming is that it can utilize various data object types referred to as classes. Previously, the `xVal` object was a single numeric value, however can analyze and work the other common data types. First R can understand the difference between an integer, a whole number, and a numeric value. The distinction is that a numeric data type can be a number with a decimal. Although this difference can seem subtle in some computational work, this has an impact. If you've been following the simple code examples in this chapter, you should have `xVal`, `newObj` and an `i` variable from the previous FOR loop. Reviewing the "Environment" pane you will note the `i` variable has a `4L` instead of just 4. This denotes that the variable is a whole number without a decimal. In contrast, the `xVal` object has a `1` without the "L." This means R is understanding this value to be a decimal or floating-point number. You can check the class difference using the `class` function applied to any object. Notice how the third `class` function call switches the returned value to "numeric" when a decimal is added.

Often this distinction is not impactful but there are times as you will learn in this book that functions expect specific object types.

```
class(i)
class(xVal)
class(i +.01)
```

In addition to integers and numeric values, common R data types include "Boolean" values known in R as "logical" object types. Boolean data types are merely TRUE or FALSE. R can interpret these values as occurring or not occurring as shown in the IF statements. Additionally, for some operations, Boolean values can be interpreted as 1 and 0 for TRUE and FALSE, respectively. For example, in R `TRUE + TRUE` will return a value of `2` while `TRUE - FALSE` will return `1`, because R interprets the Boolean as 1 − 0. Let's create a Boolean object called `TFobj` in the code below for use later.

```
TFobj <- TRUE
```

Another data type R often utilizes is a "factor." A factor is a non-unique description of information. For example, a sports team may be assigned to a conference. Another team may also be assigned to that conference as well so it is frequently a repeating value within a data set. The factor has a level, meaning the conference name, and in effect the factor level alone represents specific "meta" information such as the other teams in the conference, and even perhaps some of the team's schedule. This meta-information is inherited as a pattern within the larger data set, not explicitly defined within the object type. While this may be confusing, it will make sense eventually as the object types and classes move to multiple values instead of single values later in this chapter. The code below simply creates a single object, `teamA` with a factor defined as the Eastern conference. The function to declare value as a factor is simply `as.factor`.

```
teamA <- as.factor('Eastern_Conference')
```

In addition to factors, the last commonplace variable type includes "character." Character objects represent natural language, for example, from social media or fan forums that need to be analyzed. The field of character and string analysis is referred to as Natural Language Processing (NLP). These methods and technology underpin the popular smart speakers and voice assistants among other everyday common technologies such as e-mail spam filters. This book devotes one chapter to gauging fan engagement on a popular forum. Thus, this type of data type will be covered extensively. However, one chapter merely covers the basics of NLP and much more can be accomplished with additional methods, code, and academic literature. Below is a fictitious social media post from a fan. Character values can be declared with `as.character` but, as written here, are not necessary.

```
fanTweet <- "I love baseball"
```

In review, Table 1.2 reviews the common data types used in R and within the book. There are additional data types like `NULL` and `NA` but these are more straightforward, requiring less explanation. Once you have run all the code in the table, you can simply call `class` on each object to check that R is interpreting the object type as expected.

Table 1.2 Common R data types including integer, numeric, logical, factor, and character.

Name	Code	Description
"integer"	`x <- 5L`	A whole number without a decimal point
"numeric"	`y <- 5.123`	A floating point number

"logical"	`z <- TRUE`
	`z <- T #capital T or F`
	`is acceptable too`
		A logical "Boolean" operator either TRUE or FALSE. R will interpret TRUE as 1 and FALSE as 0 for some operations

"factor"	`playerPosition` `<- as.factor("forward")`	A factor is a distinct class often representing non-unique information. The factor classes are referred to as "levels." Here, a player position is defined as a factor with the level "forward"

"character"	`fanComment <- "I love`
	`the hot dogs at the`
	`stadium"`
		Character values, known as strings, represent natural language. Unlike factors, they can be repeating or mutually exclusive. A growing subset of analytics work includes Natural Language Processing (NLP)

Previously, the objects created such as `xVal` and `i` represented a single value. R's coding environment relies on specific data types and corresponding classes that can be more complex than a single value. For instance, R can create and work with "vectors." Vectors are merely columns of data that you may be familiar with if you're coming to R from a spreadsheets program. To create a numeric vector, you employ the combine function which is `c`. In the following code, a vector of numbers is created called `xVec`. The `xVec` object utilizes some of the objects previously created along with additional values that are explicitly declared within the `c`, combine function. Each value within the vector is separated by a comma. Once `xVec` is created, calling in the console will return multiple values where the object such as `xVal` is now substituted to their numeric equivalents.

```
xVec <- c(xVal, i, newObj, 345,678)
```

Scaling up from a single vector, one method for arranging multiple columns into a single object is with `cbind`. The `cbind` function arranges vectors in a column-wise fashion. Similarly, the `rbind` function will stack vectors as rows. The resulting object type is no longer a "numeric" or other previous type discussed, but instead "matrix" type. A matrix arranges data into rows and columns within a single object. This code creates `xMatrix` using `cbind` and simply repeating the previous vector `xVec` to create a second column. Once executed the `xMatrix` variable is in the environment and when called demonstrates a five row by two column arrangement of the data in a single object. Calling `class` on the object will return "matrix."

```
xMatrix <- cbind(xVec, xVec)
```

R has another method for arranging data as rows and columns called a data frame. The data frame object type is useful when you are working with mixed data types, for example, a player roster with names, as characters, teams as factors, statistics as numeric, and so on. All of these vectors can be organized into a single object using `data.frame`. This

Table 1.3 The constructed data frame with mixed data types.

number1	logical2	factor3	string4
1	TRUE	a	string1
4	TRUE	b	s2
1	FALSE	a	s3
345	FALSE	b	s4
678	TRUE	b	s5

code is a bit more complex because it nests functions when constructing the data frame. Within the `data.frame` function call, the first column is names "number1." It is assigned a value of `xVec` which equates to the numeric values previously constructed. The next column, "logical2," is separated by a comma and employs the `c` function combining logical values. Next, the "factor3" column is declared. This column has multiple functions including `c` to combine a vector of "a," "b," "a," "b," and "b" but then it is changed from a simple character vector to factor using `as.factor`. Finally, the fourth column, "string4," consists of various character strings. Once instantiated in the console, the `xDataFrame` object can be called to illustrate the mixed data types held within the single object. Table 1.3 shows the results of creating the `xDataFrame` object.

```
xDataFrame <- data.frame(number1 = xVec,
                         logical2 = c(T,T,F,F,T),
                         factor3 = as.factor(c('a','b','a',
                                   'b','b')),
                         string4 = c('string1', 's2', 's3',
                                   's4', 's5'))
```

R can employ either a matrix or data frame to arrange data in rows and columns. In both object types, the columns and rows must be complete. For example, you cannot `cbind` a vector with three values to another with two values. This makes the data "ragged" and for matrices r data frames requires you to fill in the cell value with NA. However, some functions require one object class over another. The difference is that a matrix must have all values be of the same data type. For example, each value in all of the columns must all be numeric or all logical. If this is not the case, the matrix function will coerce the data into characters automatically which can cause issues. As a result, most often in this text, the `data.frame` and object type are used. However, you can coerce either object type to the other using `as.matrix` or `as.data.frame` to switch. Just keep in mind the mixed data coercion mentioned previously.

The last data type discussed in this book is a "list" object. There are other object types including time series and arrays but for the most part this book employs mixed data types, with data frames and sparingly lists. If you are familiar with spreadsheets, think of a list as a "workbook" containing multiple "work sheets." Each tab of the spreadsheet programs can contain different data even single values and different types. A list is similar in that each list "element" can contain a single value, multiple values, matrices, data frames, or even more lists! The following code creates a list object with varying data types and lengths, while Figure 1.7 is a graphical representation of the list.

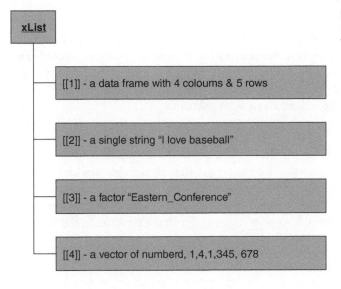

Figure 1.7 The representation of the list with varying objects.

```
xList <- list(xDataFrame,
               fanTweet,
               teamA,
               xVec)
```

In complex R objects, you can get specific sections of the data by name or through indexing. The previous list has four elements, denoted with double square brackets such as `[[2]]`. To access a specific list element, you can call the object `xList` along with its specific element index as shown below to select the fourth element, the vector of numbers.

```
xList[[4]]
```

The same can be done with matrices or data frames using single brackets. Indexing row and column data requires two inputs separated by a comma. The selection for rows is first followed by the selection for columns. For example, let's first call the `xDataFrame` object in its entirety to establish familiarity. Then select the first row and third column which represents a single cell value of the data frame. Next, you can select a different row, column combination on your own within the console to establish this single value is returned.

```
xDataFrame
xDataFrame[1,3]
```

Indexing also works for entire columns or entire rows. This is done by leaving the rows position blank or the columns position blank on either side of the comma. To call the second column of the data frame simply use single brackets, nothing on the left of the comma and a 2 to the right of the comma as shown.

```
xDataFrame[, 2]
```

Similarly, you can switch the index number to the left of the comma to obtain a specific row. Here, the entire fourth row is returned while the column position is left blank.

```
xDataFrame[4, ]
```

Besides the ability to have multiple data types, another benefit of the data frame object is the ability to declare a column by its name using the `$` sign. For example, instead of an index position the column names `$numer1` will return the entire first column of the data frame object. The two methods, indexing or by name, are equivalent but can be used interchangeably as long as the column has a declared name.

```
xDataFrame$number1
```

In fact, indexing can become more complex. You can access a specific list element, then a specific row, column, or single value by utilizing double then single brackets or `$` as shown. First, the fourth element of the list is obtained with `[[4]]`; then the second value is obtained within that vector. Keep in mind there is no need for a comma because a vector does not have rows or column. Instead, a vector merely has a position. In this case, "2" is returned.

```
# 4th element, vector 2nd position
xList[[4]][2]
```

Next, the first list element is accessed, and as a data frame, the single brackets with a comma refer to the second row.

```
# 1st element, 2nd row
xList[[1]][2,]
```

Similarly, the same data frame is indexed to return the first column because the "1" is to the right of the comma within the single square brackets.

```
# 1st element, 1st column
xList[[1]][,1]
```

Of course, you can also use both rows and column positions separated by the comma within the single brackets.

```
# 1st element, 2nd row, 1st column
xList[[1]][2,1]
```

Just to make things a bit more complex, if the list element is a data frame with named vectors, the second part of the code can employ the `$` along with the name. This will return the first list element, a data frame, and only the named column called "logical2."

```
# 1st element, named column with $
xList[[1]]$logical2
```

Lastly, since the column of this list element is being accessed, it too can be indexed. Once again, the single column does not have a row and column pairing, it only has a position. Thus, no comma is needed and only the third position is returned in this example.

```
# 1st element, names column with $, third position
xList[[1]]$logical2[3]
```

If all this seems wildly complex, do not fret. Throughout the book extensive explanation is given for both functions, inputs, and indexing. Further, with enough practice, this becomes commonplace and more readily understood.

So far, this basic explanation of R functionality has relied on base-R functions and libraries that are part of the standard installation. As mentioned previously, R can be specialized to a particular task by loading libraries. In order to obtain libraries, the `install.packages` function must be run with a package name to download the specialized functions. This is done only once per library so that the library code is installed locally to your R installation. After the download occurs you can merely call the `library` function with the name in order to enable the specialized functionality using the local installation. The code below installs a popular graphics library called "grammar of graphics" known as `ggplot2` using the `install.packages` function. After it is downloaded, the next line merely loads it as part of your R environment. This allows your R session to call functions within a "namespace" that includes base-R and now `ggplot2` functions. It serves the purpose of specializing R for improved visualizations.

```
install.packages('ggplot2')
library(ggplot2)
```

Throughout this book, multiple libraries are loaded. Novice R programmers can run into errors and frustrations regarding package installations. When executing scripts in this book that begin with `library(...)`, an error of "there is no package called ..." means you first need to use `install.packages` to download the functionality to your library. Additionally errors may occur during the `install.packages` step. This can be due to multiple reasons but most often stems from the fact that a package to be downloaded requires another package first. As a result, carefully read the console messages during the install phase to identify any other package prerequisites. If the `install.packages` function executes correctly, then it is not necessary to repeat that function for each script. Thus, the code in this book only calls `library` for each specific library enabling corresponding functionality needed for the task at hand. This assumes all libraries have been previously and successfully installed.

> To specialize R, first install a package with `install.packages` with the corresponding name. If installed without issue, simply call `library` any time your R session needs specialized functionality corresponding to the specific library. You will only need to use `install.packages` once but `library` will need to be called each time you start R and require the specialized functions of a particularly library.

In at least one instance in the book, a custom function is needed to make the code more concise. A custom function is like any other function loaded from a library. It is defined for an operation and requires an input and returns a value or object. The code below creates a simple custom function as an example. The function is declared as `plus3` with the `function` statement. Next, the input parameter is declared as `x`. This means the function will be called `plus3` and requires an input temporarily called `x`. What happens to `x` occurs within the curly brackets. In this case, a simple operation `x + 3` overwrites the internal value of 'x' and the new value is returned. The function will be an object in the environment and can accept any numeric or integer value. Here, the function is created and then applied to a value of 2. The output is assigned an object itself in 'exampleThree'.

```
plus3 <- function(x){
  x <- x + 3
  return(x)
}
exampleThree <- plus3(2)
exampleThree
```

Of course, functions can be more complex. As an example, the following function is made to be more dynamic by adding a new parameter, called 'value'. Now both are required for the function to operate. The 'x' value is now divided by the 'value' input parameter that is passed into the function. Additionally, before the result is returned from the function, the 'round' function is applied further adjusting the preceding division. In the end, for example, the custom function 'divideVal' will accept a number 5, divide it by 2, and then round the result so that it returns the value 2.

```
divideVal <- function(x, value){
  x <- x / value
  x <- round(x)
  return(x)
}
exampleValue <- divideVal(5,2)
exampleValue
```

Applying R Basics to Real Data

Let's reward your laborious work though foundational R coding with something of actual interest utilizing sports data. Like many scripts in this book, let's begin by loading packages. For each of these, you need to first run 'install.packages' and assuming that executes without error, the following library calls will specialize R for the task at hand. As an example, script using real sports data, our only goal is to obtain the data, manipulate it, and finally plot it.

To begin call 'library(RCurl)' which is a general network interface client. Functions within this library allow R to make a network connection to download the data. One could have data locally in a file, connect to an API, database, or even web scrape the data. However, in upcoming code, the data are download directly from an online repository. Next, 'library(ggplot2)' loads the grammar of graphics namespace with excellent visualization capabilities. The 'library(ggthemes)' call is a convenience library accompanying 'ggplot2' for quick, predefined aesthetics. Lastly, the 'library(tidyr)' functions are used for tidying data, which is a style of data organization that is efficient if not intuitive. Here, the basic raw will be rearranged before plotting.

```
library(RCurl)
library(ggplot2)
library(ggthemes)
library(tidyr)
```

Next, before establishing a connection between R and the data repository, a character object is created called `c1Data`. The character string is the web URL to the raw comma-separated value, CSV, file. If you open this web address in a typical browser, you will see the raw text-based statistics for regular season Dallas NBA team in the 2019–2020 season. However, the following code does not open a browser and instead downloads this simple file before loading it as an R object.

```
c1Data <- 'https://raw.githubusercontent.com/kwartler/
Practical_Sports_Analytics/main/C1_Data/2019-2020%20Dallas%20
Player%20Stats.csv'
```

Now to execute a network connection employ the `getURL` function which lies within the `RCurl` package. This function simply accepts the string URL address previously defined. Be sure to have the address exactly correct to avoid any errors.

```
nbaFile <- getURL(c1Data)
```

Finally, the base-R function `read.csv` is used with the downloaded data. The `read.csv` function is widely used because CSV files are ubiquitous. Further, the function can accept a local file path leading to a hard disk rather than the file downloaded here but the path must be exactly correct. Spaces, capitalization, and misspellings will result in cryptic and frustrating file not found errors. Assuming the web address was correct, and the `getURL` function executed without error, then the result of this code is a new object called `nbaData`. It is automatically read in as a `data.frame` object.

```
nbaData <- read.csv(text = nbaFile)
```

Unlike a spreadsheet program where you can scroll to any area of the sheet to look at the contents, R holds the data frame as an object which is an abstraction. As a result, it can be difficult to comprehend the loaded data. Thus, it is a best practice to explore the data to learn about its characteristics. In fact, exploratory data analysis, EDA, in itself is a robust field within analytics. The code below only scratches the surface of what is possible.

To being this basic EDA defines the dimensions of the data using the `dim` function applied to the `nbaData` data frame. This will print the total rows and columns for the data frame. Similar to the indexing code, the first number represents the rows and the second the columns.

```
dim(nbaData)
```

Since data frames have named columns, you may want to know what the column headers are. The base-R function `names` accepts a few types of objects and in this case will print the column names of the basketball data.

```
names(nbaData)
```

At this point you know the column names and the size of the data loaded in the environment. Another popular way to get familiar with the data is to glimpse at a portion of it. This is preferred to calling the entire object in your console. Data frames can often be tens of thousands of rows or more plus hundreds of columns. If you call a large object directly in console, your system may lag trying to print that much data as an output. Thus, the popular `head` function accepts a data object along with an integer parameter representing the number of records to print to select. Since this function call is not being assigned an object, the result is printed to console for review. The default behavior selects six though this can be adjusted for more or less observations. When called the `head` function will print the first 'n' rows of the data frame. This is in contrast to the `tail` function which will print the last 'n' rows.

```
head(nbaData, n = 6)
```

You should notice that the column `TEAM` shows "Dal" for all results in the `head` function. To ensure this data set *only* contains players from the Dallas team you can employ the `table` function specifying the `TEAM` column either by name or by index position. The `table` function merely tallies the levels or values of a column. After running the next code chunk, you see that "Dal" appears 19 times in this data set. Had there been another value in this column, additional tallied information would be presented.

```
table(nbaData$TEAM)
table(nbaData[,2])
```

Lastly, another basic EDA function is `summary`. The `summary` function can be applied to any object and will return some information determined by the type of object it receives. In the case of a data frame, the `summary` function will examine each column individually. It will denote character columns and, when declared as factor, will tally the different factor levels. Perhaps most important is how `summary` treats numeric columns. For each numeric column, the minimum, first quartile, median, mean, third quartile, and maximum are returned. If missing values are stored as "NA" in a particular column, the function will also tally that. This allows the practitioner to understand each columns range, distribution, averages, and how much of the column contains NA values.

```
summary(nbaData)
```

Now that you have a rudimentary understanding of the player level Dallas basketball data set, you can visualize aspects of it. For example, one would expect that the more minutes a player averages per game, the more points the player averages per game. To confirm this assumption, a simple scatter plot may help identify the correlation. Of course, you can calculate correlation, with the `cor` function, but often visualizing data can be a powerful tool in a sports analyst's toolkit. The `ggplot2` library contains a convenience function called `qplot` for quick plotting. This function accepts the name of a column for the *x*-axis, followed by another column name to plot on the *y*-axis. The last parameter is the data itself. The `data` parameter requires a data frame so that the specific columns can be plotted. Additionally, an optional aesthetic is added declaring the `size` for each dot in the scatterplot. The code below adds another aspect to the `qplot` to improve the overall look. Specifically, another "layer" is added from the `ggthemes` library to adjust

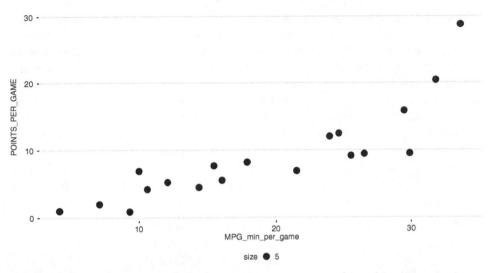

Figure 1.8 As expected the more minutes a player averages the higher the average points.

many parameters within a single function call. Here, the empty function `theme_hc` emulates the popular "Highcharts" JavaScript theme. As is standard with `ggplot2` objects, additional parameters such as aesthetics are added in layers using the `+` sign. This is not the arithmetic addition sign merely an operator to append layers to `ggplot` objects. Figure 1.8 is the result of the `qplot` and `theme_hc` adjustment using the Dallas basketball data to explore the relationship between average minutes per game and average points per game.

```
qplot(x    = MPG_min_per_game,
      y    = POINTS_PER_GAME,
      size = 5,
      data = nbaData) +
theme_hc()
```

Let's add a bit more complexity to the visualization by creating a heatmap. The heatmap chart has *x* and *y* axes but represents data amounts as color intensity. A heatmap allows the audience to comprehend complex data quickly and concisely. To begin, let's use the `data.frame` function to create a smaller data set. Here, the column names are being renamed and each individual column from the `nbaData` object is explicitly selected. The new object has the same number of rows but a subset of the columns. There are additional functions to perform this operation but this is straightforward. As the book continues, more concise though complex examples will perform the same operation.

```
smallerStats <- data.frame(player = nbaData$i.PLAYER,
                           FTA = nbaData$FTA_free_throws
                                 _attempted,
                           TWO_PA = nbaData$TWO_PA,
                           THREE_PA = nbaData$THREE_PA)
```

In order to construct a heatmap with `ggplot2`, the `smallerStats` data frame must be rearranged into a "tidy" format. This type of data organization can be difficult to comprehend for novice R programmers, but the main point is that the data is not being changed, merely rearranged. The `tidyr` library function `pivot_longer` accepts the data frame first. Next, the `cols` parameter is defined. In this case, the column to pivot upon is the `player` column. This will result in each player's name being repeated and two new columns being created. These columns are defined in the function as `names_to` and `values_to`, respectively. In the end, each player and corresponding statistic name and value are captured as a row. Whereas the `smallerStats` data frame had 19 observations with 4 columns, now the `nbaDataLong` object which has been pivoted by the `player` column has 57 rows and 3 columns. After the pivot the `head` function is executed to demonstrate the difference.

```
nbaDataLong <- pivot_longer(data = smallerStats,
                            cols = -c(player),
                            names_to = "stat",
                            values_to = "value")
head(nbaDataLong)
```

Now that the data has been modified, it will be readily accepted by the `ggplot` function. Instead of the previous `qplot` function, now the more expansive `ggplot` function is called. The first parameter is the `data` object. The next parameter is the `mapping` aesthetics. This is a multi-part input declared with yet another function `aes`. Within the `aes` function, the column names to be plotted are defined. Specifically, the *x*-axis column name, `stat`, followed by the *y*-axis column name `player`, and finally the fill value which corresponds to the `value` column. Thus, the visual is set up so that player statistics are arranged on the *x*-axis, individual players will be a single row along the *y*-axis, and the color intensity will be scaled by the players corresponding statistical value. Once the base layer plot has been defined, another layer is added with the `+` sign to declare the type of plot needed. In this case, the heatmap is called using `geom_tile`. In subsequent chapters, additional visuals are illustrated including ggplot2 and more dynamic interactive graphics. Since this text requires gray-scale graphics, another layer is added to define the color intensity between `lightgrey` and `black`. Finally, another layer is added to retitle the *x*-axis label as "Scoring Statistics" encased in quotes because it is a label not an object or column name. For simplicity, this is captured in an object called `heatPlot`.

```
heatPlot <- ggplot(data    = nbaDataLong,
                   mapping = aes(x = stat,
                                 y = player,
                                 fill = value)) +
            geom_tile() +
            scale_fill_gradient(low="lightgrey",
                                high="black") +
            xlab(label = "Scoring Statistics")
```

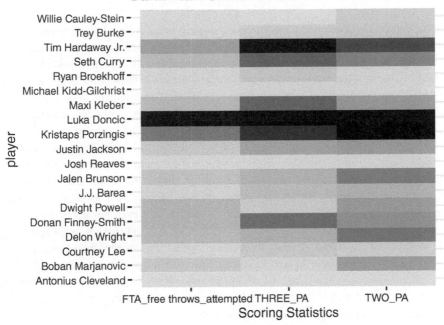

Figure 1.9 The Dallas team statistics represented in a heatmap illustrating the most impactful players among these statistics in the 2019–2020 regular NBA season.

Although calling `heatPlot` now in the console will create the visual, some additional layers can be added. First, a predefined theme for Highcharts is added, just as before using `theme_hc`. Next, a chart title is declared with `ggtitle` along with the quoted "Dallas Team Offensive Stats." Lastly, a `theme` is appended as the final layer that simply removed the legend altogether. Now when the `heatPlot` object is called, a clean, visually compelling plot is created that clearly shows the most offensively productive player for the three statistics on the team. Additionally, other player's strengths in these statistics are easily understood because their sections are darker compared to teammates. Conversely weaker players in these stats have a lighter color. These facts are more quickly understood in a visual compared to reviewing a table of player data. The result of the `heatPlot` object is shown in Figure 1.9.

```
heatPlot <- heatPlot +
  theme_hc() +
  ggtitle('Dallas Team Offensive Stats') +
  theme(legend.position = "none")
```

There are multiple ways to extend the lessons of this chapter to improve R coding fluency. For example, the data itself can be explored further or subset by position. Additional visualizations are also possible although many of these topics are covered in subsequent chapters with expanded explanations.

Positives and Negatives of R

In the end, R should be known as a scripting language. It is not a "low level language" like Java where the code itself is executed directly on the hardware such as a central processing unit, CPU. As a scripting language R cannot be compiled into an executable standalone program. As a result, R has some constraints, in that it is slower than other languages like Java and building a standalone application is not possible. However, the benefit is that R is capable of executing multiple operations borrowing from languages as needed and it well suited to statistical tasks. For example, operations in machine learning like Random Forest are called with R functions yet executed in Fortran. Still other functions borrow from C, SQL, Weka, and so on. This diversity makes the functionality high because the functional tool set is vast but with so much going on under the hood, R can be slow. Another drawback to R is that objects are stored in active memory. As a result, data objects are limited by the amount of RAM on your laptop or R-Studio server. For many data tasks this is not a problem especially as you transition to scalable cloud servers. In fact, in this text, all the data tasks and computation are relatively small. Constraints start to exist after loading millions of rows and columns in a data frame or when doing computationally complex calculations as is the case with Depp Neural Networks. However, this book is focused on sports analytics rather than big data or machine learning exclusively. Thus, these drawbacks to the R language will not be an issue.

Besides the ability to execute functions drawing from across multiple specialized languages R has other positive benefits. For example, R has a well-developed support community. Often when you are presented with an error or unknown operation, a simple online search will identify the solution. Additionally, R is optimized for statistics. Although python, a competing and more-diverse language has similar functionality, there are still differences between the two languages. For example, some machine learning-tuning parameters are better executed in R, the simple creation of dynamic HTML-based dashboards is easier or file formats like "fst" are more enhanced within R. Given that R is not picky about spacing and indentation, it is an excellent language for the novice programming. As you scale your learning in analytics and coding, you will likely want to add to your language toolkit.

Exercises

1) How is an IDE different than a coding language?

2) Describe the difference between a vector and a data frame or matrix?
   a) What is the difference between a data frame and matrix?

3) Construct a vector called `position` where the values are:
   a) "Center," "Forward," "Guard," "Forward," "Forward," and "Guard."
   b) Change the object type from character as it was constructed into a factor.

c) Tabulate the `position` factor object using `table` in a new object called `tallyPosition`.

d) Use a new function to quickly create a bar plot of the results. To do so, apply `barplot` on the `tallyPosition` object.

4) Load `library(RCurl)` then create an object called "bostonStats" by loading the file here: https://raw.githubusercontent.com/kwartler/Practical_Sports_Analytics/main/C1_Data/2019-2020%20Boston%20Player%20Stats.csv

a) How many rows does this data frame have?

b) How many columns does this data frame have?

c) Examine the last 4 rows of the data programmatically? What player is listed as the fourth from the bottom?

d) Using either indexing or column name, get summary statistics for the `GP_games_played` column. What is the third quartile of this statistic?

5) Load `library(ggplot2)` then create a quick plot of `STEALS_PER_GAME` and `TURNOVERS_PER_GAME`. Does there appear to be a relationship to the syle of play for strong defense and turnovers?

6) Load `library(tidyr)`, then create a heatmap of the Boston team data using `REBOUNDS_PER_GAME`, `ASSISTS_PER_GAME`, `STEALS_PER_GAME`, and `BLOCKS_PER_GAME` by `i.PLAYER`

a) Create a small data frame renaming the player column.

b) Pivot the data frame.

c) Create a `ggplot` visual with the pivoted data where
   i) `aes(x = stat, y = player, fill = value)`
   ii) The chart type is `geom_tile()`
   iii) The color intensity scales from "`lightgreen`" to "`darkred`"
   iv) The x-axis label "`Basketball Statistics`"

2

Data Visualization

Best Practices

Objectives

- Articulate best practices of convincing visualizations
- Understand the programmatic layering used in most popular plotting R library `ggplot2`
- Understand the difference between client and server-side data
- Create various plots with `ggplot` including sports fields and courts
- Create interactive visualizations with `echarts4r` that are client side

R Libraries

```
tidyverse
ggplot2
ggthemes
echarts4r
rbokeh
HistData
dplyr
sportyR
RCurl
```

R Functions

```
library
%>%
select
pivot_longer
mutate
ggplot
```

Sports Analytics in Practice with R, First Edition. Ted Kwartler.
© 2022 John Wiley & Sons Ltd. Published 2022 by John Wiley & Sons Ltd.

```
aes
geom_col
facet_wrap
scale_fill_manual
scale_y_sqrt
theme_void
theme
ggtitle
c
as.date
melt
geom_vline
scale_fill_brewer
theme_bw
data.frame
geom_point
theme_tufte
cor
geom_bar
as.data.frame
table
rbind
rep
coord_polar
geom_label
theme_void
rnorm
length
pie
geturl
read.csv
geom_baseball
geom_hex
theme_bw
geom_soccer
geom_basketball
geom_football
figure
ly_points
list
count
group_by
e_charts
```

```
e_bar
e_tooltip
e_title
e_y_axis
e_theme
```

Sports Context

Professional sports analysts face an uphill battle considering the domain has been run by subject matter expertise and qualitative understanding since modern professional sports teams and leagues have existed. When Michael Lewis' book *Moneyball* was published in 2003,[1] the thought of sports analytics to inform decision-making was novel. Thus, modern sports analytics in the front office is only about 20 years old compared to the hundred or so years many leagues and teams have existed. Still, organizations that rely heavily on analytics are publicly ridiculed by the likes of Charles Barkley, former professional basketball player and TV personality stating, "just because you got good stats doesn't mean you got a good team"[2] and "it's just some crap some people who were really smart made up." As with many business decisions, practical analysis is not as black and white as Charles Barkley would lead us to believe.

Although Charles Barkley and many other sports analytics naysayers have benefited from analytics outside of a sports domain in the form of logistics in e-commerce, streaming video recommendations, algorithmic trading in stocks, smart speakers, and improved search results, they judge sports as an industry as somehow unique or different. It is extremely unlikely that sports alone represent the single modern-day industry that will not benefit from quantitative analysis. In fact, this immature data fluency occurs within many industries and is not specific to sports. As with any nascent analytics application, sports analytics missteps and misguided understanding of the business objectives have led to a mistrust of the methods, giving some skeptics license to write-off technical methods in their entirety. Yet, analysis has helped teams augment player rest and practices, optimize ticket sales, and avoid poor draft picks.

On the other hand, Charles Barkley is correct noting many examples where analytics did not benefit a team. In professional sports and particularly basketball, the rosters are small, and one does not need to be an analyst to identify Lebron James or similar athlete as a super star capable of leading an otherwise mediocre roster to success. Charles Barkley neglects to note that these examples represent outlier players that are easy to identify. For teams, the economic opportunity costs regarding non-superstar or middling players may be harder to differentiate for a qualitative mindset. Thus, there is a role for both perspectives. On one hand analysis is not needed for the trained

---

1 Wikimedia Foundation. (2021, August 25). *Moneyball*. Wikipedia. Retrieved September 12, 2021, from https://en.wikipedia.org/wiki/Moneyball.

2 YouTube. (2015). *TNT's Charles Barkley rants about analytics in NBA, Houston Rockets GM Daryl Morey. YouTube.* Retrieved September 12, 2021, from https://www.youtube.com/watch?v=2asGeItzGWM&ab_channel=watchnba201415.

qualitative expert to identify obvious game strategies, business decisions, and super-stars, yet on the other hand, qualitative expertise is limited as the field of options and inputs expand.

In the end, sports decisions should be *augmented* by analytics. It is myopic to think sports decisions are exclusively qualitative or quantitative. This type of business decision-making is often referred to as "augmented intelligence" or "human over the loop" because the analysis is one factor for the human to take into consideration. It is ultimately the human that has full responsibility for the decision. Given that the cost of a data scientist[3] is less than ~5–15% of the cost of a *single* minimum professional contract[4] in a major sports league like basketball, organizations would be remiss if they did not have a single analyst on staff to supplement decisions. Avoiding a single bad contract or optimizing ticket sales could easily justify the salary expense.

To be successful, sports analytics professionals likely must work in the middle ground, acknowledging the expertise of others, data analysis as supplemental to decision-making and to set aside any intellectual arrogance often accompanying quantitative professionals. Besides excellent interpersonal communication skills, effectiveness in this scenario can be accomplished with two components. First, ensuring the analysis is part of a "data narrative." This means articulating a complete picture including the problem statement, the data used, methods, limitations, and how the outcome reinforces or deteriorates current thinking regarding the problem. It is then up to the decision maker to probe and ultimately incorporate or ignore the analysis. Despite significant effort, an analyst should not take a difference in opinion personally, their role is to supplement. The second component entails articulating the analysis in a manner fitting the audience's technical acumen. To that end, human beings have evolved superior pattern recognition capabilities.[5] According to neuroscience, superior pattern recognition or SPP is the foundation for humans' greater capacities for communication, reasoning, and abstract thought. Thus, the importance of visualization cannot be understated, particularly for non-technical audiences. Human beings are limited at grasping tabular data compared to our ability to extract meaning from patterns observed in visualizations. For example, consider the data presented in Table 2.1. It is hard to understand or interpret if a pattern is present in the 60 data points.

Yet when this data is used along with some basic plotting code shown below, a clear pattern emerges as shown in Figure 2.1.

```
library(ggplot2)
ggplot() +
  geom_point(data = allDat[31:60,],aes(x,y)) +
  geom_path(data = allDat[1:30,],aes(x,y)) +
  theme_void()
```

3 PayScale.com. (n.d.). *Average data scientist salary*. PayScale. Retrieved September 12, 2021, from https://www.payscale.com/research/US/Job=Data_Scientist/Salary.

4 Adams, L. (2021, August 5). *NBA minimum salaries for 2021/22*. Hoops Rumors. Retrieved September 12, 2021, from https://www.hoopsrumors.com/2021/08/nba-minimum-salaries-for-2021-22.html.

5 Mattson M. P. (2014). Superior pattern processing is the essence of the evolved human brain. *Frontiers in neuroscience*, *8*, 265. https://doi.org/10.3389/fnins.2014.00265.

Table 2.1 Sixty seemingly unrelated data points.

x	Y	x	Y
1.5	−1	0.9375	−0.75
1.48831028	−0.8925148	0.92287778	−0.7098258
1.45378771	−0.7900554	0.88585301	−0.6884495
1.39804653	−0.6974129	0.84375	−0.6958734
1.32369314	−0.618919	0.81626921	−0.7286237
1.23420422	−0.558244	0.81626921	−0.7713763
1.13376417	−0.518225	0.84375	−0.8041266
1.02706945	−0.5007333	0.88585301	−0.8115505
0.919109	−0.5065867	0.92287778	−0.7901742
0.81493092	−0.5355116	0.9375	−0.75
0.71940647	−0.5861555	1.1875	−0.75
0.63700225	−0.6561503	1.17287778	−0.7098258
0.57157141	−0.7422231	1.13585301	−0.6884495
0.52617341	−0.8403492	1.09375	−0.6958734
0.50293102	−0.9459405	1.06626921	−0.7286237
0.50293102	−1.0540595	1.06626921	−0.7713763
0.52617341	−1.1596508	1.09375	−0.8041266
0.57157141	−1.2577769	1.13585301	−0.8115505
0.63700225	−1.3438497	1.17287778	−0.7901742
0.71940647	−1.4138445	1.1875	−0.75
0.81493092	−1.4644884	1.0625	−1.25
0.919109	−1.4934133	1.04787778	−1.2098258
1.02706945	−1.4992667	1.01085301	−1.1884495
1.13376417	−1.481775	0.96875	−1.1958734
1.23420422	−1.441756	0.94126921	−1.2286237
1.32369314	−1.381081	0.94126921	−1.2713763
1.39804653	−1.3025871	0.96875	−1.3041266
1.45378771	−1.2099446	1.01085301	−1.3115505
1.48831028	−1.1074852	1.04787778	−1.2901742
1.5	−1	1.0625	−1.25

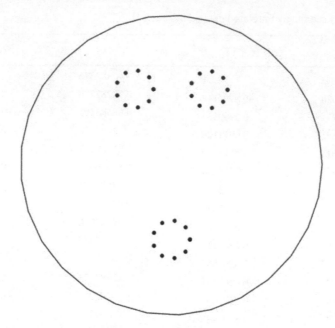

Figure 2.1 The plots displayed with a path and points showing a clear recognizable face pattern.

   The reader's brain can probably identify a basic face within this plot while it is likely very few if any readers were able to note this pattern from tabular data alone. The abstract pattern is reasoned once the data has been visualized and is made even easier to interpret with the choice to use both `geom_point` and `geom_path` for separate sections of the data. Had the decision been made to use only individual points, the pattern may be more difficult to identify. Thus, visualizations are as much practitioner choice as much as the data itself and care must be taken to avoid misleading the audience. For an audience, the power of visualization is noteworthy. As a result, this chapter is devoted to best practices and code foundations used throughout the book. It is worth mentioning that some of the methods cited here are useful in other domains beyond sports analytics such as medicine, government policy making, and business visualizations.

Plotting Best Practices and Static Images

This chapter purposefully has basic code explanations compared to other chapters. Visual best practices are shared, and code is illustrated primarily for reconstruction, encouraging thoughtful reflection about the visual not necessarily the code functionality or the analytical meaning which is purposefully simplistic.

Let's begin by learning about one of the most famous visual analytics professionals in history, Florence Nightingale. Interestingly, Florence Nightingale is considered a hero of modern medicine and nursing not just statistics and visualization. In fact, she worked tirelessly during the Crimean War supporting British troops. Known as the "Lady with the Lamp," she advocated for improved hospital conditions and came to be known as a social reformer.[6] However, one of her uncanny abilities was to convince others with less data literacy to agree with her data-driven observations. For example, she noted a decline in mortality rates among soldiers when cleanliness was improved in patient care. As a result, she is also regarded not only as a stalwart in nursing and social reformer but also a statistician with masterful powers of persuasive visualizations.

The Crimean War occurred from October 1853 to February 1856. It was a large war including Russia, France, the United Kingdom, and the Ottoman Empire. The war itself was described as "notoriously incompetent butchery."[7] Making matters worse were appalling hospital conditions including dirty water where a horse had died near the source, thereby contaminating it, lack of ventilation in the hospital, and preventable deaths from communicable diseases regarded as "unavoidable." Florence Nightingale advocated for sanitation and to support her aims, tracked patient outcomes before and after sanitation standards were implemented.

According to Tim Harford's podcast regarding Florence Nightingale,[8] "Florence Nightingale was not only a nurse she was also ... a total nerd." Harford states she was the first female fellow of the Royal Statistical Society and "...a master of data visualization." In the podcast, she is credited with saying "whenever I am infuriated [by reluctance to accept data], I avenge myself with a new diagram," demonstrating her belief that visualizations help others understand and make data useful in a broad context. In her journey documented in the podcast, a takeaway is that well-constructed plots help inform decisions.

One of her most renowned visuals includes the "Nightingale Rose." It is a temporal comparison of deaths by type and month with a before and after contextualization. Figure 2.2 is the original Rose diagram. Nightingale's goal was to articulate the significant drop in mortality before sanitation on the right and after on the left. The audience's first impression is that the overall area is much larger when conditions were abhorrent. Next, the "disease" death type represented in the outermost section shrinks after sanitation leaving the categories "other" and "wounds" to be a higher proportion of the overall deaths in any specific month. Lastly, it appears as though the "other" and "wounds" sections have a relatively stable existence appearing in almost all months regardless of cleanliness while "disease" is largely absent after hygiene protocols are enacted. The audience is expected to understand that deaths decreased significantly. Further, the subsection within deaths labeled "disease" decreased the most so the audience is meant to intuit that these types of

6 History.com Editors. (2009, November 9). *Florence Nightingale*. History.com. Retrieved September 13, 2021, from https://www.history.com/topics/womens-history/florence-nightingale-1#:~:text=Florence%20Nightingale%20(1820%2D1910),the%20founder%20of%20modern%20nursing.

7 Troubetzkoy, A. S. (2006). *A brief history of the Crimean War: The causes and consequences of a medieval conflict fought in a modern age*. Robinson.

8 Harford, T. (2021, April 16). *Cautionary tales – florence nightingale and her geeks declare war on death*. Tim Harford. Retrieved September 13, 2021, from https://timharford.com/2021/03/cautionary-tales-florence-nightingale-and-her-geeks-declare-war-on-death.

deaths are avoidable. At the time, Figure 2.2 was attention getting and consumable for non-data fluent audiences. The intent and conclusion were clear and unquestionable.

To reconstruct the Rose diagram, considering the following `ggplot` code directly from Neil Saunders blog post[9] (containing extensive code explanations for those readers that are interested). Overall, the code employs "tidy" principles used sparingly in this book but is concise in this plot construction. The code selects specific columns and pivots to a "tidy" format before creating new variables to group the pre- and post-data. Finally, the familiar `ggplot` layer instantiates the bar charts. To mimic the "rose" aspect of the data, a layer `coord_polar` is appended making the plot coordinates become anchors around a pole. The resulting reconstruction is shown in Figure 2.3.

```
Nightingale %>%
  select(Date, Month, Year, contains("rate")) %>%
  pivot_longer(cols = 4:6, names_to = "Cause", values_to =
  "Rate") %>%
  mutate(Cause = gsub(".rate", "", Cause),
         period = ifelse(Date <= as.Date("1855-03-01"),
"April 1854 to March 1855", "April 1855 to March 1856"),
         Month = fct_relevel(Month, "Jul", "Aug", "Sep", "Oct",
"Nov", "Dec", "Jan", "Feb", "Mar", "Apr", "May", "Jun")) %>%
```

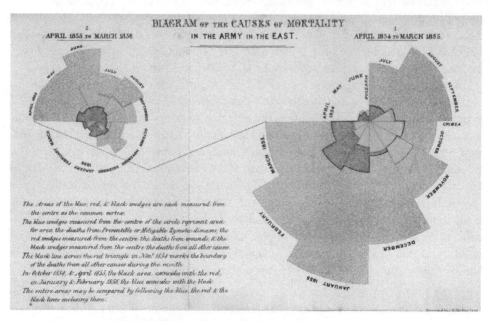

Figure 2.2 The "Nightingale Rose Diagram" visualizing a stunning improvement to patient outcomes once sanitation was instantiated.

---

9 SAUNDERS, N. (2021, March 18). *Florence Nightingale's "Rose charts" (and others) in GGPLOT2*. What You're Doing Is Rather Desperate. Retrieved September 14, 2021, from https://nsaunders.wordpress.com/2021/03/16/florence-nightingales-rose-charts-and-others-in-ggplot2.

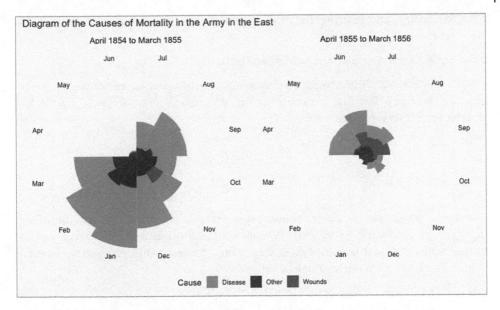

Figure 2.3 The original Nightingale Rose chart reconstructed in ggplot.

```
ggplot(aes(Month, Rate)) +
geom_col(aes(fill = Cause), width = 1, position = "identity") +
coord_polar() +
facet_wrap(~period) +
scale_fill_manual(values = c("skyblue3", "grey30", "firebrick")) +
scale_y_sqrt() +
theme_void() +
theme(axis.text.x = element_text(size = 9),
      strip.text = element_text(size = 11),
      legend.position = "bottom",
      plot.background = element_rect(fill = alpha
      ("cornsilk", 0.5)),
      plot.margin = unit(c(10, 10, 10, 10), "pt"),
      plot.title = element_text(vjust = 5)) +
      ggtitle("Diagram of the Causes of Mortality in the
Army in the East")
```

By today's standards, the Nightingale Rose diagram is not considered best practice but was among the first infographics and is noteworthy as a result. The layout makes tracking month-to-month changes difficult to compare. Code chunks are below to recreate the data visualization in a more contemporary understanding of visualization practices for comparison. First, select only specific columns within the square brackets to create `florence`.

```
florence <- Nightingale[,c('Date', 'Month', 'Year',
                           'Disease.rate',
                           'Wounds.rate', 'Other.rate')]
```

Next, to help `ggplot` interpret the *x*-axis, declare the `Date` column as a date class with `as.Date`.

```
florence$Date <- as.Date(florence$Date)
```

Here, `reshape2`'s `melt` function is shown as an alternative to the previous `pivot_longer` function. The first parameter is the `florence` data, followed by the key variables and then value pair vectors.

```
florence <- melt(florence,
                 id.vars       = c("Date", "Month"),
                 measure.vars = c("Disease.rate",
                                  "Wounds.rate", "Other.rate"))
```

Instead of a polarized bar chart, the entire temporal relationship is shown in the following `ggplot` code using `geom_col`. A single vertical line is added with `geom_vline` to denote the pre- and post-aspects of sanitation. The last two layers simply improve aesthetics. Figure 2.4 is the resulting bar chart.

```
ggplot(florence, aes(Date, value)) +
  geom_col(aes(fill = variable), color = 'black', position =
"identity") +
  geom_vline(xintercept =
               as.numeric(florence$Date[grep('1855-03-01',
florence$Date)])) +
  scale_fill_brewer(type = "seq", palette = "Greys") +
  theme_bw()
```

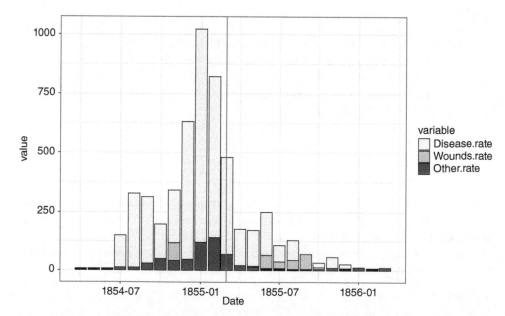

Figure 2.4 The Nightingale data replotted as a bar chart making temporal comparisons easier.

Interestingly, when viewed in this manner, the data presents a less compelling narrative for sanitation. It is clear the overall death did go down so sanitation did have an impact. However, when one can more easily track the data month to month, the drop off in "Disease" rates begins before proper sanitation and even increases over previous months in some instances. The outcome is still the same though less pronounced in the original format. Thus, care must be taken to not purposefully mislead the audience. It is evident that practitioner design choices will impact the data narrative understood by the audience.

Another visualization expert within the modern day is Edward Tufte. In this various works, courses, and speeches, he mentions six best practices[10] elucidated below. In fact, there is a `ggthemes` library predefined style called `theme_tufte` to easily add his visual best practices. His six best practices are shown as follows:

- Show comparisons: Contextualize with known or easily understood subject matter
- Use multivariate data: Every *relevant* type of information should be included
- Establish credibility with the audience: Include source information in a presentation
- Show causality: Allow the human to infer causality and encourage a takeaway
- Integrated modality: Careful integration of text and images
- Focus content: Minimizing the chart architecture wherever possible and avoid "chart junk"

In addition to the overall best practices briefly described above, care must be taken for choosing specific plot types. There are many types of charts overall and illustrated throughout this book. However, the two most common are scatter and bar charts. A scatter plot usually features two variables plotted in *x* and *y*-axes. According to the American Society for Quality (ASQ), a scatter plot is to be used when the data has paired numerical information and/or there is an independent and dependent relationship between the two data vectors.[11] Further, ASQ states a scatter plot is useful when a data pair relationship is suspected and can be additionally helpful to identify root causes.

Consider the following partial US Paralympic Swimming Roster from the 2020 Paralympic Game built in code below. The `swimmers` data frame represents eight athletes with `height`, `weight`, and `gender` columns.

```
athlete <- c('Cailin Currie','Colleen Young','Elizabeth Marks',
             'Hannah Aspden','Jessica Long','Evan Austin',
             'Rudolph Garcia-Tolson','Robert Griswold')
height <- c(67, 68, 65, 70, 69, 73, 73, 72)
weight <- c(130, 135, 125, 130, 140, 175, 137, 155)
gender <- c('F', 'F', 'F', 'F', 'F', 'M', 'M','M')
swimmers <- data.frame(athlete, height, weight, gender)
```

A scatter plot can help identify the relationship between height and weight. The following code uses `ggplot` to instantiate the plot with the *x*-axis as `height` and the *y*-axis

---

10 Tufte, E. (n.d.). *Six fundamental principles of design - tufte on design and Data*. Google Sites. Retrieved September 14, 2021, from https://sites.google.com/site/tufteondesign/home/six-fundamental-principles-of-design.

11 American Society for Quality. (n.d.). *What is a scatter diagram?* ASQ. Retrieved September 1, 2021, from https://asq.org/quality-resources/scatter-diagram.

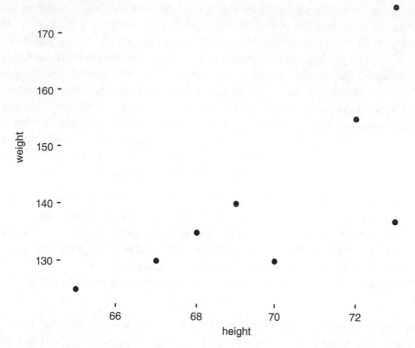

Figure 2.5 The Tufte inspired scatter plot, demonstrating a positive relationship between height and weight among Paralympic swimmers.

as `weight`. Next, the `geom_point` layer adds the points followed by the Tufte inspired aesthetics layer `theme_tufte`. The result is shown in Figure 2.5.

```
ggplot(swimmers, aes(height, weight)) +
  geom_point() +
  theme_tufte()
```

One could argue that the positive relationship between the value pairs could be noted with a correlation measure. This is easy using the `cor` function as shown here which will return a correlation of 0.72.

```
cor(swimmers$height, swimmers$weight)
```

However, data can be more complex than a linear relationship. This could result in a correlation that is 0 yet a visual representation could still help identify a noteworthy pattern. For example, ponder the fake data constructed in `fakeData` with `data.frame`.

```
fakeData <- data.frame(x = c(-2,-1,0, 1,2,3,4),
                       y = c(5,0,-3,-4,-3,0,5))
```

Calling `cor` on this data will result in a value of 0. Thus, without proper visualization, one could mistakenly believe there is no relationship. This is exemplified below.

```
cor(fakeData$x,fakeData$y)
```

However another `ggplot` with this data illustrates a pattern that the summary correlation function missed. The human brain is still able to identify the pattern despite the correlation not identifying the nonlinear relationship. Admittedly, there are other mathematical evaluations, usually less well known, that will identify a nonlinear relationship shown in the following scatter plot, Figure 2.6, for example, alternating conditional expectations from the `acepack` package.

```
ggplot(fakeData, aes(x, y)) +
  geom_point() +
  theme_tufte()
```

Another common chart type is the bar chart. In a basic bar chart values are represented as rectangles. The area of the rectangle increases as the value increases making basic bar charts good for comparing quantities between discrete categories. An example basic bar chart can be constructed using `geom_bar` in the below code. Notice, the `aes` argument only has a single input, `gender`. The code automatically will tally according to the single variable `gender`.

```
ggplot(swimmers, aes(gender)) +
  geom_bar() +
  theme_tufte()
```

Similarly, when the data object already has tallies or values for illustration, the layer `geom_col` can be employed. Here, a simple tabulation is performed, then switched to a `data.frame`. Now the `ggplot` `aes` input has two variables as *x* and *y*, respectively. This is a requirement of using `geom_col` because the tally is not automatically applied by group as is the case with `geom_bar`. Either code will construct similar bar charts shown in Figure 2.7.

```
tally <- as.data.frame(table(swimmers$gender))
ggplot(tally, aes(Var1, Freq)) +
  geom_col() +
  theme_tufte()
```

Next, let's construct a side-by-side bar chart. This type of bar chart is useful for comparing subsection values across categories. First, let's add a partial Paralympic Cyclist roster to the `swimmer` data from before. Once again, the variables `name`, `height`, `weight`, and `gender` are manually constructed. Then, a new column `sport` is constructed to track each athlete competition.

```
athlete <- c('Oksana Masters', 'Jamie Whitmore', 'Chris Murphy',
             'Joe Berenyi', 'Alicia Dana',
             'Freddie De Los Santos', 'Jill Walsh')
height <- c(68, 65, 72, 69, 67, 71, 66)
weight <- c(122, 112, 155, 160, 105, 150, 128)
gender <- c('F', 'F', 'M', 'M', 'F', 'M', 'F')
cyclists <- data.frame(athlete, height, weight, gender)

bothRosters <- rbind(swimmers, cyclists)
```

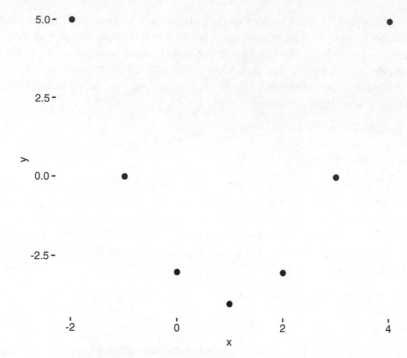

Figure 2.6 The Tufte inspired, nonlinear scatter plot. A human can easily identify two relationships within the data, descending to point [1,−4].

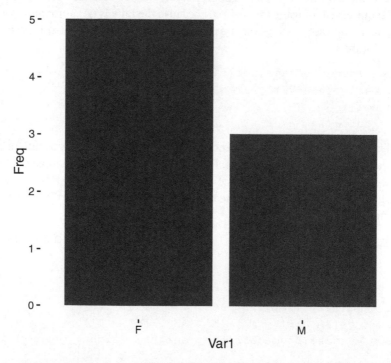

Figure 2.7 The basic bar chart showing the example data had more female athletes than male.

```
bothRosters$sport <- c(rep('swimming', nrow(swimmers)),
                       rep('cycling', nrow(cyclists)))
```

Once the data has been appended in the new object `bothRosters`, the following code creates a black and grey side-by-side bar chart. The challenging part for new R programmers is the `geom_bar` layer input. Elsewhere in the book, the `stat = "identity"` input dictates the layer should not automatically tabulate the data. In this example, the data needs to be tabulated so it is not included. However, to get the bar side by side, the parameter `position = "dodge"` is included followed by aesthetics. Figure 2.8 is the resulting bar chart showing a tallied comparison intersecting both `gender` and `sport`.

```
ggplot(bothRosters, aes(x=sport, fill=gender)) +
  geom_bar(position='dodge') +
  theme_tufte() +
  scale_fill_manual(values = c("grey30","grey90"))
```

Another common plot type is the stacked bar chart. In side-by-side bar charts, it is difficult for the audience to sense the totals of the major categories. In the previous figure, the total values for cycling or swimming are hard to determine. If the goal of the visualization is to compare proportions within a category, then a stacked bar chart will suffice. The code is almost the exact same as previous but the `position` parameter has been removed. The result is Figure 2.9 which clearly shows the total number of swimmers is more than cyclists. Additionally, the subsection of males is equal, and the audience can easily understand the difference occurs with female athletes in the abridged roster data.

```
ggplot(bothRosters, aes(x=sport, fill=gender)) +
  geom_bar() +
  theme_tufte() +
  scale_fill_manual(values = c("grey30","grey90"))
```

The last common bar chart is the proportional stacked bar chart. A proportional stacked bar chart is helpful when there are differences in magnitude among categories. This type of chart lets you compare proportions of subsections across the categories without losing sight of any very small categories. Another three athletes are added manually in the following code to construct the `crew` data frame. It is then row-bound to the other rosters with `rbind` to make `allRosters`.

```
athlete <- c('Blake Haxton','Danielle Hansen', 'Laura Goodkind')
height  <- c(38, 73, 67)
weight  <- c(150, 160, 148)
gender  <- c('M', 'F', 'F')
sport   <- rep('rowing', 3)
crew    <- data.frame(athlete, height, weight, gender, sport)

allRosters <- rbind(bothRosters, crew)
```

If one were to construct the previous bar charts with `allRosters`, the proportion within a category becomes hard to interpret for the rowing cohort because it is significantly smaller than the other sports in the data. This is especially problematic when a subsection of the data is extremely underrepresented. The following code illustrates how

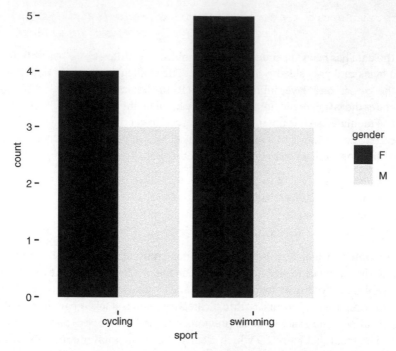

Figure 2.8 The side-by-side bar chart lets the use compare more dimensions of the data across categories. For example, one can easily compare female cyclist values to female swimming.

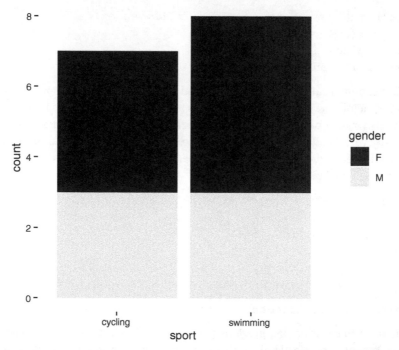

Figure 2.9 The stacked bar chart demonstrating the overall difference in totals stemming from the female cohort.

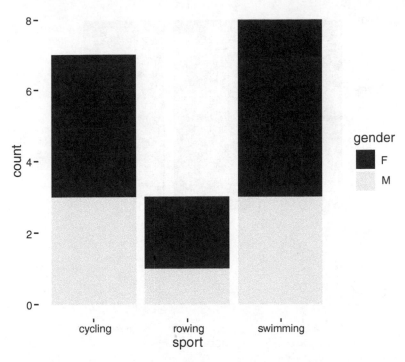

Figure 2.10 Since the tally of rowing is less than the other sports, comparing the proportionality of the gender variable across sports is difficult.

a bar chart makes comparisons hard when there are underrepresented values. Figure 2.10 reconstructs a stacked bar chart using similar code to the previous plot. This view makes the proportionality of gender more difficult to compare between sports. With this small example data it is still possible to interpret but more realistically the data with huge imbalances would make it impossible such as a bar chart representing thousands of data points alongside another category with only a few dozen.

```
ggplot(allRosters, aes(x=sport, fill=gender)) +
  geom_bar() +
  theme_tufte() +
  scale_fill_manual(values = c("grey30","grey90"))
```

Instead, a proportional stacked bar chart will help the audience understand this proportionality information more readily. The following code has an additional input in `geom_bar`. The `position = "fill"` parameter denotes that the bar will fill the plot and be calculated as a portion. The bars are expected to fill the visualization space. Now the proportion of gender is easily understood regardless of the total number of athletes in each sport. This is illustrated in Figure 2.11.

```
ggplot(allRosters, aes(x=sport, fill=gender)) +
  geom_bar(position="fill") +
  theme_tufte() +
  scale_fill_manual(values = c("grey30","grey90"))
```

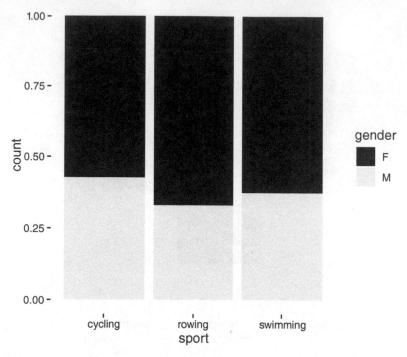

Figure 2.11 The proportional stacked bar chart showing that the proportion of gender Paralympic athletes within rowing is similar to the other sports regardless of the total number of athletes in each sport.

Although not shown in these examples for simplicity's sake, additional data dimensionality may be added to improve a plot's narrative. For example, a third data dimension can be added to a scatter plot by color coding the points, changing their shape according to a factor, or adjusting the size or transparency of a point based on a continuous variable. Using the original `swimmers` data, the additional data dimension of `gender` can be incorporated by shape and a legend. Keep in mind, additional data dimensions are not exclusive to scatter plots. Additionally, if the analysis does not naturally intersect the new dimension(s), the new variables can be considered "chart junk" according to Tufte. Still, the code below adds an additional aesthetics within the `geom_point` layer declaring `shape` as the `factor` class vector `gender` as an example of adding a third contextual dimension. Figure 2.12 shows that not only there is a relationship between height and weight but the added context that males athletes are both taller and heavier in this simplified data set.

```
ggplot(swimmers, aes(height, weight)) +
  geom_point(aes(shape = factor(gender))) +
  theme_tufte()
```

Generally, too many dimensions may overwhelm an audience so Tufte's "Focus Content" best practice should be considered. Throughout the book, additional data dimensions are utilized beyond the basic examples shown previously. Table 2.2 summarizes common chart types regardless of dimensionality which is more context driven.

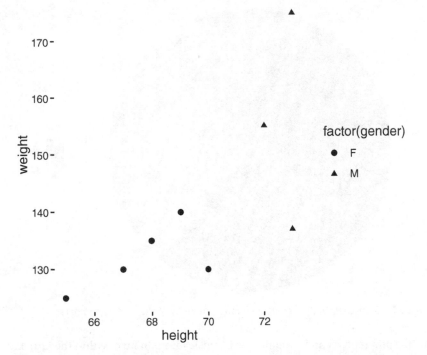

Figure 2.12 The swimmer data showing three dimensions of data in the scatter plot, height, weight, and gender.

Table 2.2 A summary of the types of bar charts and when to use them.

Chart type	When to use
Scatter plot	To identify a relationship between paired data
Basic bar chart	Comparing quantities or frequencies
Side-by-side chart	Comparing subsection values *across* categories
Stacked bar chart	Compare proportions *within* a category
Proportion stacked bar chart	Compare proportions of subsections across the categories

So far, this chapter has focused on best practices, two very common chart types and when to use them. Entire books and curricula have been built expanding upon these foundation introductions. In contrast the next section describes two popular yet over used chart types. This section represents the reverse, bad charts and how they should be avoided.

Some online blogs go as far as to say "Pie Charts Suck."[12] While blunt, pie charts are widely regarded as bad form. Common sense states a pie chart *should* be useful to compare values across categories. However, comparing a lot of pie slices and discerning

---

12 Quach, A. (2017, August 23). *Why pie charts often suck*. Medium. Retrieved September 16, 2021, from https://medium.com/the-mission/to-pie-charts-3b1f57bcb34a.

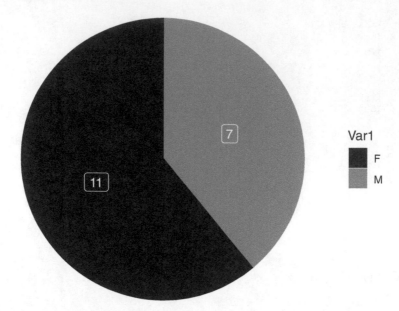

Figure 2.13 An acceptable pie chart given the simplicity of the underlying data.

subtle pie differences can be tough or even misleading. In fact, within the `ggplot` official documentation, it is noted that "polar coordinates have major perceptual problems
... use with EXTREME caution."[13] Here is some code that tallies the genders for comparison among all sports within a pie chart. First, `table` and `as.data.frame` are used
to tabulate the `gender` variable.

```
genderTally <- as.data.frame(table(allRosters$gender))
```

Next the `ggplot` is instantiated, and values are explicit so the `geom_col` layer creates a bar chart. However, the `coord_polar` layer rotates the bars into a polarized
coordinate system creating the pie chart. The remaining layers add aesthetics. The resulting Figure 2.13 is an acceptable comparative visualization based on the code.

```
ggplot(genderTally, aes(x = "", y = Freq, fill = Var1)) +
  geom_col() +
  coord_polar(theta = "y") +
  geom_label(aes(label = Freq),
             color = "white",
             position = position_stack(vjust = 0.5),
             show.legend = FALSE) +
  theme_void() +
  scale_fill_manual(values = c("grey30","grey50"))
```

Unlike the other types of bar charts which can still help the audience understand
data within, across, and proportionally, the pie chart is limited as complexity increases.
Here is some code with untallied data recreating the previous stacked bar chart. The

13 Wickham, H. (2021, June 25). *Polar coordinates - coord_polar.* - coord_polar • ggplot2. Retrieved
September 16, 2021, from https://ggplot2.tidyverse.org/reference/coord_polar.html?q=polar.

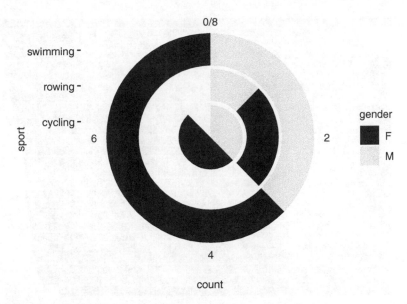

Figure 2.14 The identical data portrayed in a nearly nonsensical pie chart.

only addition is the `coord_polar` layer. Simply adding this layer turns an otherwise useful stacked bar chart into an incomprehensible pie chart! Compare Figure 2.14, a hard to interpret pie chart, with the same data, and nearly identical code portrayed as a stacked bar chart to understand the difference in usefulness.

```
ggplot(allRosters, aes(x=sport, fill=gender)) +
  geom_bar() +
  theme_tufte() +
  scale_fill_manual(values = c("grey30","grey90")) +
  coord_polar(theta = "y")
```

Even if the data for the pie chart is organized appropriately, with many pie slices, it is difficult for the audience to discern. Let's construct some fictitious data and order is in ascending value.

```
set.seed(1234)
vals <- rnorm(length(letters), 10,0.5)
badPie <- data.frame(letters = letters,
                     value = vals)
badPie <- badPie[order(badPie$value),]
```

First, let's construct a bar chart and orient the bars horizontally which is easier for the eye to track with many categories.[14] Like previous code, `ggplot` is instantiated. Next, the columns are added with `geom_col` while the next two layers are aesthetic choices. The last layer orients the plot with `coord_flip`. In Figure 2.15, the fictitious category "t" is the highest value while "d" is the least and other comparisons can be made.

```
ggplot(badPie, aes(x=reorder(letters, value), value)) +
```

14 Quach, A. (2017, August 23). *Why pie charts often suck*. Medium. Retrieved September 16, 2021, from https://medium.com/the-mission/to-pie-charts-3b1f57bcb34a.

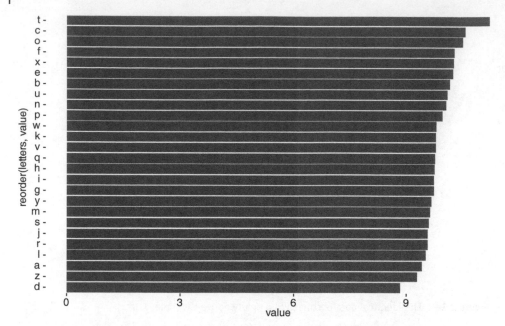

Figure 2.15 Even with many similar value categories, a bar chart allows for comparisons.

```
geom_col() +
theme_tufte() +
scale_fill_manual(values = c("grey30","grey90")) +
coord_flip()
```

Switching to a pie chart and plotting the data is much more problematic. Here, the base-R "pie" function is used. The first input includes the plot value, while the next is the slice labels followed by a chart title. In contrast, to the previous plot, Figure 2.16 has too many slices to make easy comparisons. In fact, the audience is left to assume the slices are all equal which differs from the flipped bar chart.

```
pie(badPie$value, labels = letters, main="Base Pie Chart")
```

At best, a pie chart performs similarly to the most basic bar chart and in other multidimensional data sets should be avoided. With simple data, a pie chart has equal usefulness to a bar chart but has inferior utility in all other aspects as the data complexity grows. Thus, just avoid a pie chart and use a bar chart in almost all cases.

Another discouraged chart type includes three-dimensional (3D) charts. Here is an example from Wikimedia.[15] Figure 2.17 shows a basic 3D bar chart. 3D charts are often visual clutter resulting in a confused audience. Since extra color devoted to each bar to add the appearance of the z dimension, that is not supported by data, the bars seem swollen or exaggerated. For example, looking closely at Figure 2.17, a bar's front edge may be at ~0.75, while its trailing edge is closer to 1.0. Thus, the exact value is hard to discern. Similarly, 3D pie charts are very exaggerative as some slices have the additional z-dimension

---

15 Wikimedia. (n.d.). *KChart-screenshot2*. Wikimedia is a global movement whose mission is to bring free educational content to the world. Retrieved September 15, 2021, from https://commons.wikimedia. org/wiki/Category:Vertical_3D_bar_charts#/media/File:KChart-screenshot2.png.

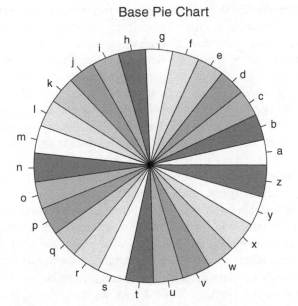

Figure 2.16 A complicated pie chart where the audience cannot discern differences.

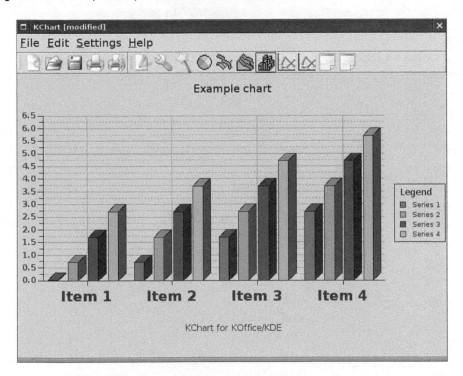

Figure 2.17 A basic 3D bar chart example.

appearance which makes the slice appear larger merely for appearance but not supported in data. Further, 3D pie charts are not technically circles which makes comparisons difficult. However, R has some interactive plotting where an audience member could interact with an x–y–z dimensional plot, such as a scatter plot where points are in 3D space. These charts differ in that the z dimension is supported by a data dimension but even their utility is limited causing more effort for the audience to interact with the plot. Mostly 3D charts contain "chart junk" and likely should be minimized or avoided altogether.

Clearly this chapter is only scratching the surface of visual possibilities. As a sports book, it is important to demonstrate the `ggplot` manner to plot various fields, courts, and pitches. Other chapters use these visuals in context, particularly baseball's geospatial chapter. The following section should serve as a reference for the practitioner applying book concepts across sports. Ross Drucker's package ` sportyR` is the easiest method to plot various sports arenas. The upcoming sports arena visuals follow the package's official documentation with some basic changes. Interestingly, not only can the package plot static geospatial sports images, with `gganimate` short animations of player or ball movement can be constructed. According to the library documentation the library provides multiple options even within sports based on collegiate, professional, or international dimensional changes. Table 2.3 shows the court options as of version

Table 2.3 The robust sportyR package arena options from the official documentation.

Sport	League	Primary plotting unit
Baseball	MLB	ft
Basketball	FIBA	m
Basketball	NBA	ft
Basketball	NCAA Basketball	ft
Basketball	WNBA	ft
Football	CFL	yd
Football	NCAA Football	yd
Football	NFL	yd
Hockey	IIHF	m
Hockey	NCAA Hockey	ft
Hockey	NHL	ft
Hockey	NWHL	ft
Soccer	FIFA	m
Soccer	MLS	m
Soccer	NCAA Soccer	m
Soccer	NWSL	m
Soccer	Premier League	m
Tennis	ITF	ft
Tennis	NCAA	ft

1.0.3.[16] Currently, the package code includes "Plot made via sportyR" as a caption which could be considered "chart junk." However, it is likely to be removed in subsequent library releases. In the meantime, one way to remove this caption is to crop images or to clone the package and adjust the hidden function which adds the caption by calling the code below to see the caption parameters and rewrite the function and then rebuild the package.

```
getAnywhere(create_plot_base)
```

Creating a baseball diamond instantiated in `ggplot` is simple with a single code line shown below.

```
geom_baseball('mlb')
```

Adding data to the base layer is easily by adding a new layer with data declared. A hexbin layer is added, and for the sake of publishing, the color is filled as `grey` and the background theme changed to `theme_bw`. However, in color graphics these should be omitted to visualize the density within bins by color. The reduced color visual is shown in Figure 2.18.

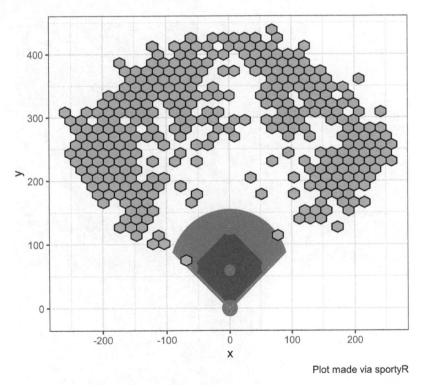

Plot made via sportyR

Figure 2.18   An example ggplot baseball diamond.

16 Drucker, R. (2021, April 20). *Plot scaled 'Ggplot' representations of sports playing surfaces [R package sportyr version 1.0.1]*. The Comprehensive R Archive Network. Retrieved September 16, 2021, from https://cran.r-project.org/web/packages/sportyR/index.html.

```
geom_baseball('mlb') +
   geom_hex(data = baseballHits,
            aes(x = x, y = y),
            color = 1, fill = 'grey') +
   theme_bw()
```

Similarly, a soccer pitch is instantiated with `geom_soccer` and some additional parameters depending on the league.

```
geom_soccer('ncaa')
```

There are additional parameters for plotting half courts in all `sportyR` visuals except for the baseball diamond. Next, half a professional court is instantiated along with a rotation. The data points plot the *x–y* coordinates for Matthew Dellavedova's 2018 and 2019 assists as an example. The data is obtained with a URL string passed to `getURL`; then it is overwritten with `read.csv`. Next, the basketball court is called with parameters as discussed. Finally, the data points are added with `geom_point`. The result is shown in Figure 2.19.

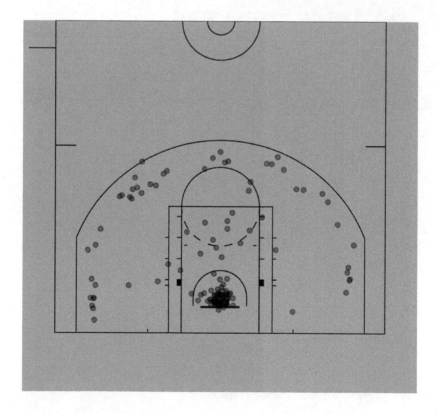

Plot made via sportyR

Figure 2.19 A basketball court with example assist data from Cleveland Cavalier's Matthew Dellavedova's 2018/19 season.

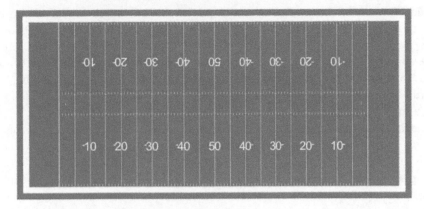

Plot made via sportyR

Figure 2.20 A basic professional football field with grey instead of green color.

```
dellavedova <- 'https://raw.githubusercontent.com/kwartler/
Practical_Sports_Analytics/main/C2_Data/Dellavedova_18_19_
season.csv'
dellavedova <- getURL(dellavedova)
dellavedova <- read.csv(text = dellavedova)
geom_basketball('nba', full_surf = F, rotate = T) +
  geom_point(data = dellavedova,
             aes(x = original_x,
                 y = original_y),
             alpha = 0.5)
```

One can also change the base layer color easily. Here is a professional football field dimension with a grey background for easier publishing but the color could be changed to any hexadecimal value. The function `geom_football` merely needs the parameter `grass_color` to be adjusted. A similar adjustment can be made within `geom_basketball` with the parameter `court_paramer_color`. The basic football field with an adjusted background is shown in Figure 2.20.

```
geom_football('nfl', grass_color = '#808080')
```

The package documentation is robust with additional aesthetic parameters. Readers are encouraged to review the official documentation if the elementary preceding examples do not suffice or want to plot other sports arenas like hockey which are not covered herein.

Interactive Plots

Now that you have a good grasp of static visuals which can be saved as "jpeg" or "png" formats among others, an interesting and useful way for an audience to understand a data narrative is through user interaction. R has multiple packages that support the construction of lightweight javascript and HTML-based plots allowing a user to zoom or hover

over data for more context. Although the https://www.htmlwidgets.org has a robust gallery and multiple packages listed supporting this type of user interaction, the book primarily demonstrates dynamic plotting with two packages `rbokeh` and `echarts4r`.

The conceptual construction of both dynamic packages mimics `ggpplot`. However instead of the addition sign, these packages use the pipe forwarding operator, `%>%`. Regardless of the package, the same best practices should be applied. In the following code, a simple scatter plot is constructed using `rbokeh`.

To begin a base bokeh layer is created with `figure`. Another layer is added using `ly_points` to instantiate the actual data which includes *x* and *y* axis column names followed by the data object. As an example, the `color` and `glyph` parameters are referring to existing column names while the `hover` parameter dictates a user interaction and specific columns. In the screenshot captured in Figure 2.21 user interaction and controls are shown. In Figure 2.21, the user's mouse is hovering over an athlete and a tooltip is shown alerting the user to the athlete and sport. On the right side, there are user interaction icons for zooming, panning resetting, and even saving a static image from the dynamic plot. Later in the book, more dimensions and complexity are added to bokeh plots. This is merely an example, so the reader understands the difference between static and dynamic plots.

```
figure() %>%
   ly_points(height, weight, data = allRosters,
             color = gender, glyph = gender,
             hover = list(athlete, sport))
```

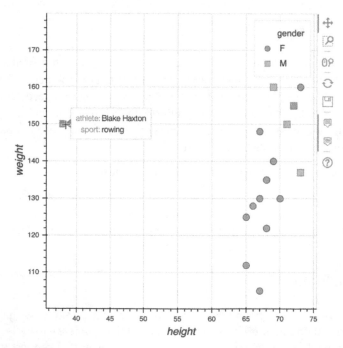

Figure 2.21   An example `rbokeh` scatter plot based on a screenshot demonstrating the tooltip user functionality.

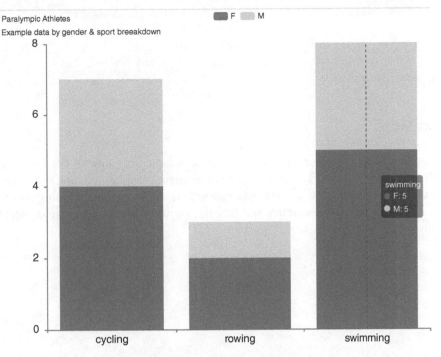

Figure 2.22 The `echarts4r` stacked bar chart with tooltip.

Another JavaScript visualization package, John Coene's package `echarts4r`, has many functions, and predefined themes used throughout the book. The book examples use many more layers and advanced construction methods than the basic example below. In this elementary code, the first line forwards the `allRosters` table to a summary function from `dplyr` called `count`. The function will tally the records by the sport and gender columns. As recommended by the package author, this is sent in a grouped manner using both `group_by` and the pipe operator, `%>%`. This example constructs a simple stacked bar plot defined in `e_charts` defining the *x*-axis with the `sport` column and the additional parameter `stack="grp"`. Next, the new `n` variable is added within `e_bar`. Lastly, layers improving user interaction and aesthetics are added. The subsequent chapters elucidate beyond this example, but it is shown here to improve reader familiarity with upcoming code and as a reference. Subsequent uses show additional user interaction like zooming and saving as a static image. The resulting stacked bar plot in Figure 2.22 has been screen shot to show the user's interaction in another tooltip.

```
allRosters %>% count(sport, gender) %>% group_by(gender) %>%
  e_charts(sport, stack = "grp") %>%
  e_bar(n) %>%
  e_tooltip(trigger = "axis") %>%
  e_title(text = "Paralympic Athletes",
```

```
            subtext = "Example data by gender & sport
                    breeakdown") %>%
    e_y_axis(splitArea = list(show = F),
            splitLine = list(show = F)) %>%
    e_theme('gray')
```

Next Steps

Subsequent chapters provide not only basic understanding of analytics but also a means to visualize the output for a data narrative. For example, machine-learning approaches in upcoming chapters provide visuals and explanations in the hopes of winning over skeptics. Remember the data narrative and intuitive comprehension will increase adoption within organizations with data-skepticism.

3

Geospatial Data

Understanding Changing Baseball Player Behavior

Objectives

- Download baseball data from various sources
- Perform a "crosswalk" inner-join with data to append additional information
- Chart a player's performance over time
- Web scrape player data from a GET request
- Tabulate pitch types by year
- Visualize the change by pitch type over time
- Create and interpret a box plot of pitch speed by type and time
- Create a 2D density plot of pitch type
- Make JavaScript interactive and static plots for each visual in this chapter

R Libraries

```
Lahman
ggplot2
ggthemes
echarts4r
dplyr
RCurl
rvest
lubridate
tidyr
rbokeh
remotes
```
—*See installation of github packages below*.

This chapter introduces unofficial package loading. In addition to the tens of thousands of official R packages shared on CRAN, many developers create and maintain their own. Often these packages are developed using the version control website www.github.com.

One method for installing unofficial packages is with the `remotes` package. Once loaded, you can call `install_github` and pass in the username and package repository. Here, the user name "BillPetti" and package "baseballr" are called. Next, user "bayesball" and "CalledStrike" are declared. At the time of writing both packages are supported and provide significant functionality for exploring baseball data. As a backup, the book's repository provides `baseballr_0.8.4.tar.gz` and `CalledStrike_0.5.6.tar.gz` files for local installation without the need for the `remotes` package. This may also be needed in case the functionality demonstrated in this chapter changes within the unofficial packages.

```
library(remotes)
install_github("BillPetti/baseballr")
install_github("bayesball/CalledStrike")
```

If successful, you can simply load the libraries as any other package using the `library` function as shown below.

```
library(CalledStrike)
library(baseballr)
```

R Functions

```
library
<-
getURL
read.csv
head
table
intersect
left_join
subset
paste
ggplot
aes
geom_point
geom_line
ggtitle
theme_hc
theme
as.factor
%>%
e_chart
e_line
e_toolbox_feature
e_theme
e_tooltip
```

```
e_title
paste0
read_html
html_table
nchar
make.names
as.Date
year
as.data.frame.matrix
t
prop.table
round
data.frame
pivot_longer
group_by
summarize
geom_boxplot
facet_grid
grepl
!
with
order
list
unique
e_connect_group
e_arrange
collect_player
location_compare
geom_density_2d_filled
add_zone
xlim
ylim
coord_equal
figure
ly_cret
ly_hexbin
split
lapply
function
grid_plot
swing_plot
rbind
is.na
as.data.frame
names
c
```

Sports Context

Professional US baseball has installed high-speed-tracking cameras in all ball parks. The system is called "Statcast" and it generates a massive amount of baseball data that was unthinkable years ago. The types of statistics are almost overwhelming with pitching attributes like velocity and spin rate alongside hitting data like launch angle and distance. For players not pitching or hitting, the Statcast system also tracks sprint speed and even arm strength of fielders. Each of these and more are tracked play by play but also can be linked by player or team to understand never-before elements of the game over time.

According to www.mlb.com, even the shortened 60 game season of 2020 generated 260,000 pitches and 43,000 batted balls resulting in a robust set of data points.[1] With so much data coupled with a historically statistically minded fanbase, this trove of information represents a new era for both fan and professional.

This chapter exposes the reader to the basics of obtaining data, visualizing and hopefully extracting meaningful player insights. The first step illustrates the various methods to obtain the data, followed by down-selecting to a single player. Overall, this chapter should aid in data manipulation and thinking robustly about the temporal and spatial nature of data. For instance, the data is subset to a player, then a statistic reviewed at the seasonal level. Later, the Statcast data is obtained, and individual pitch types are tabulated by season along with seasonal comparison of velocity and type. Finally, geospatial pitch and swing location are examined. This chapter serves as a foundation for thinking systemically when presented with relatively large data sets where periodicity and other factors can impact outcomes. Novice analysts may struggle with the magnitude and variation within the data but this chapter should help to identify initial inquires laying a foundation for truly novel insights.

Today's modern organization does not evaluate opportunities solely on Statcast data but in collaboration with qualitative and external inputs for a data-driven decision. The reason being is that player selection, evaluation, and game lineups are high impact where costs for mistakes can be immense financially. For example, reviewing pitch data alone does not help a talent scout when the player may have a substance abuse problem or be in need of a surgery. Data-driven decisions like these are considered "human over the loop." In human over the loop data-driven decision-making, "the person supervises the system and can intervene."[2] While this perspective may be novel in machine learning implementations or automated decision systems, the inclusion of human perspective is well documented in fields such as education and psychology where surveys, journal reviews, and micro-ethnographies compliment collected data to create a holistic perspective not siloed in attributes of the collected data.[3] This chapter's data primarily focuses on pitch types,

---

1 Major League Baseball. (n.d.). *Statcast: Glossary*. MLB.com. https://www.mlb.com/glossary/statcast.

2 Khatry, S. (2020, September 11). *The Feedback Loop: How Humility in AI Impacts Decision Systems*. The Feedback Loop How Humility in AI Impacts Decision Systems. https://www.datarobot.com/blog/the-feedback-loop-how-humility-in-ai-impacts-decision-systems.

3 Johnson, T. (1993). *PMEEP: Does It Creep into the Worldview of Participants? Microethnography Inquiry in Progress*. Washington, DC: National Science Foundation. (ERIC Document Reproduction Service No. ED 356 972).

spatial location of pitches as the ball crosses the plate, and spatial location of a batter when contact has been made along with an additional dimension of exit velocity meaning the speed the ball comes off the bat. For this spatial data, the x–z coordinates are visualized for comparisons by season and player. The importance and meaning of these comparisons is up to the human evaluator or plot audience; hence, the exercise is a "human over the loop" decision where one can incorporate externalities to enhance meaning.

For reference, the pitch classifications from Statcast are shared in the following:

- AB Automatic Ball
- AS Automatic Strike
- CH Change-up
- CU Curveball
- EP Eephus
- FC Cutter
- FF Four-Seam Fastball
- FO Forkball
- FS Splitter
- FT Two-Seam Fastball (synonymous with SI)
- GY Gyroball
- IN Intentional Ball
- KC Knuckle Curve
- KN Knuckleball
- NP No Pitch
- PO Pitchout
- SC Screwball
- SI Sinker (synonymous with FT)
- SL Slider
- UN Unknown

Code

As always in the text's scripts, load the libraries to specialize the R instance. Our intent is to download dynamic data from the Major League Baseball, MLB, site, manipulate it, and create player level visualizations to understand behaviors. The first library `Lahman` has predefined data objects as part of the package. This data will be used before accessing more dynamic, up-to-date data from the Internet.

```
# libraries
library(Lahman) #seasonal data
library(ggplot2)
library(ggthemes)
library(echarts4r)
library(dplyr)
library(RCurl)
library(rvest)
```

```
library(lubridate)
library(tidyr)
library(rbokeh)
library(remotes)
library(CalledStrike)
library(baseballr)
```

Often package authors do have internal data objects for examples and sometimes as references for use with functions. The `Lahman` package includes data frames for the latter. In either case, simply call the function `data` after loading the library to access the specific object. Technically, the R environment creates a "promise" which is a declared path representing the data object. However, practically the object can be called without any distinction. The object is loaded into active memory from the "promise" once the object name is employed in code. In case packages are updated and data formats are changed, both objects are included in the book's repository so the script can still be executed without revision. In that case, additional work will be needed to update the scripts after this chapter's core concepts are learned.

```
data("People")
data("Pitching")
```

Next, load a cross-walk file. Many times, in data science and analysis, you have unique identifiers with data in one table but need to have data in another table appended to the first. For example, the second table may have the same unique keys as the first yet a different set of columns. As a result, various joins may be required to match the data according to the identifier or shared column. Business analysts that are familiar with spreadsheet programs perform a similar option across sheets with "v-lookup" and "h-lookup." Frequently in practice these additional tables are referred to as cross-walks. The code below accesses a cross-walk file using `getURL` along with `read.csv`. Since Mac, Windows, and Linux operating systems differ slightly, sometimes an unparsed character appears ahead of the first column's name. The `names` function is applied to the object along with the square bracket `1` to rename the first column explicitly. The entire operation is on the left of the assignment operator though depending on your operating system may not be needed. However, in the interest of robust coding, this operation ensures consistency for later table joins no matter the operating system.

```
xWalkFile <- 'https://raw.githubusercontent.com/kwartler/Prac-
tical_Sports_Analytics/main/c3_Data/lahman_mlb_xWalk.csv'
xWalkFile       <- getURL(xWalkFile)
xWalk           <- read.csv(text = xWalkFile)
names(xWalk)[1] <- 'IDPLAYER'
```

Let's get familiar with the three data objects by calling `head` on each object. Note the `People` object has a `playerID` column with birth, death (if applicable), height, weight, batting, throwing handedness, and professional baseball starting and ending (if applicable) career dates. This data set contains more than 20,000 professional players dating back to 1871. The `Pitching` data table contains the `playerID` column but different data specific to pitchers. The second data frame contains seasonal team, league, and pitching statistics. The `People` data frame has one entry for a player because aspects like "height" and "weight" do not change. In contrast, the `Pitching` data frame has multiple rows with the same `playerID` because an athlete may, and often does, play for multiple teams throughout a career. The one-to-many table relationship for players is frequently observed in other domains such as a customer with a single address placing multiple orders recorded in another table. Lastly, reviewing the `xWalk` object has some additional distinct player level information from a subset of the entire player population. Specifically of interest, another identification column called `MLBID`.

```
head(People)
head(Pitching)
head(xWalk)
```

Examining a Single Pitcher Analytically

Now let's search for a specific pitcher to begin the analysis. First, declare strings for a player's first and last name. Updating these strings as standalone objects makes code updates easier compared to explicitly declaring first and last names multiple times throughout the script. This code creates two string objects called `playerFirst` and `playerLast`, respectively.

```
playerFirst <- 'Miguel'
playerLast  <- 'Castro'
```

Using the player name objects, apply a `grep` command on each specific column `nameLast` and `nameFirst`. The `grep` function is a pattern-matching command that returns the index position, like a row number, when a pattern is found at least once. The `grep` function is often employed in natural language processing to quickly scan for words in large documents using "regular expression" syntax. The `grep` function accepts a string to search for then a character vector to search within. In fact, "regular expressions" can be nuanced and useful beyond this simple demonstration. The function returns row numbers corresponding to the character vector where a match was identified. Specifically these `grep` functions will return the all row numbers where "Miguel" is found and another vector of numbers wherever "Castro" was found in the respective columns.

```
firstIdx <- grep(playerFirst, People$nameFirst)
lastIdx  <- grep(playerLast, People$nameLast)
```

Table 3.1 is a simplistic example employing `grep`. Table 3.1 is an abridged subset of the `People` data frame. Using `grep` with "Lou" and searching the `nameFirst` column returns the integer `2` because that is where the pattern was found. Similarly applying the `grep` command with "Whitaker" on the `nameLast` column would return both `c(2,3)` in Table 3.0 because the pattern was found in both rows.

Keep in mind the code creating `firstIdx` and `lastIdx` is searching more than 20,000 records.

Table 3.1 An abridged `People` data frame demonstrating the usefulness of `grep`.

playerID	birthState	...	nameFirst	nameLast
whistle01	MO	...	Lew	Whistler
whitalo01	NY	...	*Lou*	*Whitaker*
whitapa01	MO	...	Pat	*Whitaker*

At this point, both `firstIdx` and `lastIdx` contain all instances of "Miguel" and "Castro" for their individual columns. However, the analysis requires a single player named "Miguel Castro." Thus, the `intersect` function is employed to identify the specific numbers shared between the two objects. The code below creates the final `index` object to select a single player from among the 20,000. In the previous example using Table 3.1, the intersection of `2` and `c(2,3)` is obviously `2` which is the single player "Lou Whitaker" represented as the second row.

```
index <- intersect(firstIdx, lastIdx)
```

The result of the `intersect` function above is the single number 2933. This represents the single player row for "Miguel Castro." When the `index` object contains more than one number as is often the case with common names, a manual review is needed to ensure the correct single player row number is selected. This can be achieved by reviewing the date of birth or other player data to narrow down the selection. However, this code example returns a single row so no manual review is necessary.

Once the single row is identified, the `index` object is used within square brackets to select the single row of interest within `People`. The new object is called `onePlayer`. Table 3.2 is a condensed data frame for the specific player "Miguel Castro" obtained using `grep` and `intersect` between the two columns.

```
onePlayer <- People[index, ]
```

To append additional data to this specific one row data frame a "left-join" will be performed from the `dplyr` package. There are various join types which primarily add columns from one table to another using one or more unique keys though there are other joins that do not append data. As shown in gray in Figure 3.1, all records in the left data frame "A" are retained. Any records that share an identifier between the "A" and "B" data frames are selected. For these specific records, the information in data frame "B" is appended as new columns. This portion of the data is symbolized as the overlapping section between the circles. For left-joins, records in data frame "B" that do not share an identifier with "A" are dropped. This is symbolized in Figure 3.1 as the non-shaded portion. As previously stated, all records in "A" are retained but any records that are not

Table 3.2 The single row for Miguel Castro player information.

playerID	nameFirst	nameLast	...	bats	throws	retroID	debut
castrmi01	Miguel	Castro	...	R	R	castm002	2015-04-06

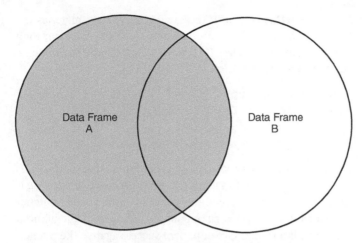

Figure 3.1 Conceptually demonstrating a left join between two data frames.

shared between the two tables will get "NA" values for the new columns appended from "B." This is represented as the left most half-moon gray section in Figure 3.1. In the upcoming code, note the number of columns in `onePlayer` is 26. After the left-join, the data frame is wider, with the additional information from the `xWalk` data frame. Now the `onePlayer` object has 32 columns.

Now that you know the mechanics of the left-join, let's unpack the code parameters. The `left_join` function accepts a pair of data frames, "A" and "B," respectively. Optionally, the `by` declaration identifies which column(s) are shared as unique identifiers. In this code, the columns differ slightly as an example. The `onePlayer` column `playerID` is equivalent to the `xWalk` column `IDPLAYER`. This parameter is technically optional because the `left_join` function will identify shared columns automatically *if* the names are identical.

> Although the `left_join` can automatically identify shared columns by name, it is a best practice to use the `by` parameter. Automatic identification can lead to unintended joins when multiple columns are simultaneously used as keys because each unique combination will represent a unique key identifier.

```
onePlayer <- left_join(onePlayer, xWalk,
                       by = c( 'playerID' = 'IDPLAYER'))
```

The `onePlayer` object now has some duplicative columns such as `birthdate` from the original `onePlayer` derived from `People` and `BIRTHDATE` from the `xWalk`. While it is good practice to remove these duplicates before or after the join, the code can ignore them because the point of the join is to specifically append the official `MLBID` which will be used later.

Next, use the `subset` function to filter the `Pitching` data frame for specific years and the player in question, "Miguel Castro" corresponding to playerID "castrmi01." The code chunk below first accepts the `Pitching` data frame and then multiple logical conditions. The first condition is whether or not `Pitching$playerID` matches the `onePlayer$playerID` followed by another condition when `yearID` is greater than 2015 and finally again if `yearID` is less than 2020. If all three logical conditions evaluate to TRUE, the row(s) are returned from `Pitching`.

```
seasonalPitcher <- subset(Pitching,
                   playerID == onePlayer$playerID &
                   yearID > 2015 &
                   yearID < 2020)
```

The new object `seasonalPitcher` has seasonal information such as `teamID`, `W`ins, `L`osses, and `G`ames for four seasons. A foundational metric in baseball pitching is the earned run average, ERA. The ERA represents the number of earned runs a pitcher allows per nine innings. Earned runs are defined as opponents runs that occur without the aid of a fielding error. Since this is a measure of opponent success against the pitcher, lower is better. Using `ggplot` let's plot a simple line chart to understand Miguel Castro's ERA consistency. First, declare a string title for the upcoming charts within the object `chartTitle`. The `paste` function simply concatenates any objects as character strings. The function utilizes the `playerFirst` and `playerLast` objects rather than an explicit and duplicative declaration. This helps by having only a single place in the code to edit when changing between players.

```
chartTitle <- paste(playerFirst, playerLast, "stats over time")
```

To create the visualization first pass in the data `seasonalPitcher`. Next, declare the aesthetics with `x` and `y` variables. One of sometimes confusing aspects of `ggplot` line charts is the need for a grouping variable. For line charts data points are connected and sometimes there is a grouping variable which can be declared if there are multiple line series. However, since this is a single line chart series representing a single player, the group can be declared as `grouping = 1`. The next layer adds default `geom_points` as if constructing a scatterplot. The next layer adds the line series with `geom_line`. Lastly, both `ggtitle` and `theme_hc` add some predefined aesthetics. The `chartTitle` declared earlier is used as the string parameter within the title layer. The resulting figure is demonstrated in Figure 3.2.

```
ggplot(data=seasonalPitcher,
       aes(x=yearID, y=ERA, group = 1)) +
  geom_point() +
  geom_line() +
  ggtitle(chartTitle) +
  theme_hc()
```

Throughout the book, the `echarts4r` package is also employed so the visuals can be interactive JavaScript. The following code recreates Figure 3.2 using this method. First, while `yearID` is an integer, it needs to be declared as a factor. This aids the `e_chart` function accept the data as discrete classes not continuous numbers.

```
seasonalPitcher$yearID <- as.factor(seasonalPitcher$yearID)
```

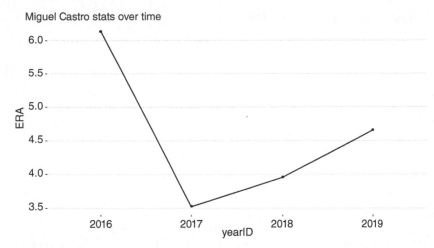

Figure 3.2 Miguel Castro's ERA which has been deteriorating from 2017 to 2020.

The `e_chart` function is similar to the base layer function `ggplot`, whereby additional layers are added in succession. First, the `e_line` layer is added along with the column names `yearID` which is accepted as the *x*-axis. Again, similarly to `ggplot` and other "tidy" libraries, there is no need to add the data frame with `$` and column name. The following layer declares the line with `e_line` while specifying the *y*-axis column name deriving the values. The `e_toolbox_feature` with the `feature = "saveAsImage"` parameter adds a small icon in the plot letting the user download the plot as a static "portable network graphic, PNG." Finally, the layers `e_theme`, `e_tooltip`, and `e_title` add simple aesthetics including the chart title with `chartTitle`. In contrast to `ggplot`, the layers are added with the pipe-forwarding operator `%>%` and the visual itself is interactive. As a user's mouse pointer passes over a point, a "tooltip" will appear with the specific value.

```
seasonalPitcher %>%
  e_chart(yearID) %>%
  e_line(ERA) %>%
  e_toolbox_feature(feature = "saveAsImage") %>%
  e_theme('gray') %>%
  e_tooltip() %>%
  e_title(chartTitle)
```

Figure 3.3 is the PNG output of the JavaScript line chart constructed with `echarts4r`.

At the time of writing, the www.mlb.com website provides "Statcast" data through the Internet. The site utilizes its own identification key which is why the `left_join` was performed previously. This joined the `playerID` value to its corresponding `MLBID` value. With this information R can easily load and web scrape a player's information hosted at the MLB website. To make the code robust with fewer places to edit, the URL construction is performed with the `paste0` function as opposed to being explicitly declared when player inquiries change. The `paste` and `paste0` functions concatenate

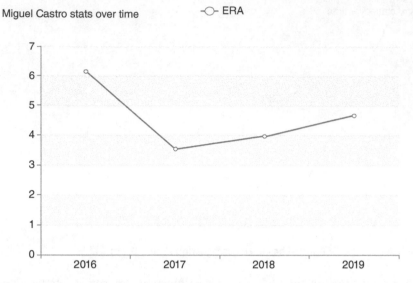

Figure 3.3 The PNG export of the `echarts4r` visual showing Miguel Castro's seasonal ERA.

inputs into a string. The difference is that `paste0` does so without a space between the string inputs. Additionally, noncharacter inputs will be coerced to characters with these functions. Here, the base section of the URL is a string and it is appended to the `onePlayer$MLBID` column value.

```
statsURL <- paste0('https://baseballsavant.mlb.com/statcast_
search?player_type=pitcher&type=details&player_id=',onePlayer
$MLBID)
```

Load this URL into any web browser to see the data in question. If it loads without an error, the data is ready to be collected. The `rvest` package is a convenient package to "haRVEST" web data. It is a port of the popular python package "beautiful soup." The first step is to use `read_html` to open a headless browser, one without a graphical user interface front end. This allows R to load and retain the raw HTML. In case the MLB backend data formatting or URLs change a copy of this data, object has been saved to the book's repository.

```
pitches <- read_html(statsURL)
```

> Keep in mind that the web scraping is dynamic, and the manuscript was written while the 2021 season was still underway. This may result in some 2021 statistics differing than is shown in subsequent code.

Once the HTML document is downloaded as an R object, the needed information is extracted into a typical R data frame for analysis. Similar to `echarts4r`, the `rvest` package author prefers the use of the pipe `%>%` operator to forward object for additional manipulation. The following code forwards the `pitches` HTML document to the `html_table` function. This function parses the HTML table into a data frame. Many web-scraping efforts are more complicated because the data is not in a simple table so there is a need to select specific sections and perform additional manipulations. However, this web page is simple because it populates more aesthetically pleasing and complicated visualizations on the MLB site most fans see when viewing the MLB pages. The returned object is a list yet only the first element is needed. As a result, the double bracket `[[1]]` is used to declare `pitchStats` object.

```
pitches     <- pitches %>% html_table()
pitchStats <- pitches[[1]]
```

The resulting data frame has a column `Pitch` with an assigned code for what type of pitch was identified using ball-tracking cameras deployed during professional games. However, some of the pitches in the data set are blank. One method to remove the rows with blank values is by applying `nchar` to the column as shown below. The `nchar` function returns an integer representing the number of characters in a character object. It is vectorized so will return a row-wise vector of values. The statement is logically evaluated to return `TRUE` if the number of characters is *greater than* zero. This evaluation is performed to the left of the comma which represents an evaluation applied to rows. In contrast, logical evaluations to the right of the comma would be applied to columns. Remember the goal is to retain the rows where the `Pitch` column is blank so the evaluation is to the left of the comma. All of this is nested within the `pitchStats` data frame with single brackets. After running the code, the data frame is reduced in size from its original row count.

```
pitchStats <- pitchStats[nchar(pitchStats$Pitch)>0,]
```

Since the data is from an HTML page, the column names may be inappropriate for use in R. For example, column names starting with or containing special characters can be troublesome when coding. Thus, the following code simply redeclares the column names to text that is more convenient to work with. On the left of the assignment operator the `names(pitchStats)` is declared on the right side with `make.names` applied to the existing column names again using `names`. While it can be confusing to describe the code itself is straightforward. The `names` function obtains the existing column headers. The `make.names` function creates "syntactically valid names out of character vectors. The first six rows are reviewed using the `head` function merely as a convenience considering the various manipulations after downloading the HTML.

```
names(pitchStats) <- make.names(names(pitchStats))
head(pitchStats)
```

The data review illustrates the `Date` column which can be used for this chapter's annual analysis. R can interpret dates as an object class with the `as.Date` function applied to the column. This function accepts a character object and will coerce it to a date class. Sometimes there are reasons to declare the format of the string positions representing months, days, and years or other temporal increments. However, in this example, the data is unambiguous and is therefore recognized without the format parameter. After the data frame column class is changed, the lubridate package function `year` is used to extract only the year from the original date. This result of the `year` function is declared in a new column to the left of the assignment operator called `pitchStats$year`.

```
pitchStats$Date <- as.Date(pitchStats$Date)
pitchStats$year <- year(pitchStats$Date)
```

The next step is to tabulate the pitch type by year. The R-base `table` function counts factor levels and is capable of performing cross-classifying tabulation. In this case, `table` cross-tabulates the `pitchStats$Pitch` column by the `pitchStats$year` column. This entire expression is nested in `as.data.frame.matrix`. The `table` returns a contingency table, an object of class "table" not data frame making additional manipulation and use difficult. The `as.data.frame.matrix` function checks if an object is a data frame and if it is not will attempt to coerce it to one. Table 3.3 is an abbreviated table of the `pitchTypes` data frame.

```
pitchTypes <- as.data.frame.matrix(table(pitchStats$Pitch, pitch
Stats$year))
```

Instead of raw count of pitch types, it can be useful to review the data as a proportion of either the row or column. In this particular use case, the review is performed by columns representing years. Thus, the `prop.table` function accepts a matrix object and then performs a proportional calculation according to the `margin` parameter. The `margin` declaration can either be a `1` for proportions calculated as rows or a `2` for column-wise proportions. For example, the column-wise proportion will take the 2015 year column shown in Figure 3.2. It calculates the sum of the column which is 293. Each individual value in the column is then divided by the column sum. For example, 49 "CH" pitches divided by 293 total pitches in 2015 is 16%. Similarly, 174 "FF" pitches divided by 293 is 59%. Thus, the sum of all percentages is 1 representing the total proportion of pitches for the year. This calculation illustrates the proportional mix of pitch type by year regardless of the pitcher's total number of games, innings, or even pitches. The entire proportional table is then transposed using base-R's `t` function. Next, the values are rounded to three decimals by passing the matrix to the `round` function with the number of rounded digits parameter. Table 3.4 shows the transformation to floating point numbers and rounded operation as a proportion of the column along with the transposition so that pitch types are now column headers.

```
pitchProps <- t(prop.table(as.matrix(pitchTypes), margin = 2))
pitchProps <- round(pitchProps, 3)
```

Table 3.3 Miguel Castro's year-over-year pitch type tally by year.

	2015	2016	2017	...	2020
CH	49	13	108	...	89
FF	174	136	19	...	0
IN	6	0	0	...	0
SI	0	618	852	...	238
SL	64	91	285	...	148

Table 3.4 Miguel Castros' pitch type by year as a proportion of pitches for each year.

	CH	FF	IN	SI	SL
2015	0.167	0.594	0.02	0.000	0.218
2016	0.054	0.567	0.000	0.000	0.379
2017	0.105	0.018	0.000	0.600	0.277
2018	0.152	0.001	0.000	0.584	0.262
2019	0.200	0.000	0.000	0.489	0.311
2020	0.187	0.000	0.000	0.501	0.312
2021	0.263	0.000	0.000	0.435	0.302

Next, let's declare `pitchProps` as a `data.frame` object with a specific column for year rather than a row attribute. The new column name is `yr`.

```
pitchProps <- data.frame(pitchProps, yr = rownames(pitchProps))
```

For easy plotting in `ggplot2`, the data can be pivoted to the long format. The `tidyr` library's `pivot_longer` function increases the number of rows while decreasing the number of columns. The function does not change the data merely its orientation. The first input is the data parameter. Next, the columns to be pivoted into the long format are declared. True to "tidy-verse" packages, column name inputs do not need quotations. In subsequent code chunk, all columns except `yr` will be pivoted to long format. The `yr` column is excluded because the `yr` text in the code parameter is preceded by a minus sign. The `names_to` parameter accepts the key column name which is stated as "stat." The final parameter is the `values_to` input representing the corresponding value for each key-value pairing. In the end, each key-value pair *for each year* is returned in a triplet style data object. While the explanations in this section of this chapter may seem trying, the code execution is concise, and the explanations are meant to aid learning more so than merely copy pasting code snippets. Table 3.5 shows the first six rows of the manipulated data. Notice the values themselves did not change.

Table 3.5 The reorientation of the pitch data to the long format.

Yr	Stat	Value
2015	CH	0.167
2015	FF	0.594
2015	IN	0.02
2015	SI	0.00
2015	SL	0.218
2016	CH	0.054
...	...	...

```
pitchPropsLong <- pivot_longer(data      = pitchProps,
                               cols      = -c(yr),
                               names_to  = "stat",
                               values_to = "value")
```

Using the longer format data a line chart by pitch type may illustrate a change in the player's approach which may contribute to the ERA change observed earlier. First, the `chartTitle` is redefined using the `playerFirst` and `playerLast` objects with a different string description. This is used within the `ggtitle` layer in the visualization code. Specifically, the base layer `ggplot` function accepts the long format data `pitch-PropsLong` with the aesthetics defined as a parameter. Within the `aes` the x-axis is defined as `yr`, the y-axis as `value`, the grouping is declared as `stat`, and finally the line type is adjusted by the `stat` column with `linetype`. This is optional but aids color-blind audiences or black and white publications. The next layer defined the plot type as a line chart using `geom_line`. Within this layer, the code can declare the color grouping using `aes(color=stat)`. The two final layers add `ggtitle` and a predefined theme from high charts using `theme_hc`. Figure 3.4 shows that the pitch type "FF" was highly used until the 2016 season but was replaced within the player's efforts with the "SI" type. The "SL" remained constant as a proportion of the player's repertoire and "CH" saw a slight increase.

```
chartTitle <- paste(playerFirst, playerLast, "pitch type over
time")
ggplot(pitchPropsLong,
       aes(x = yr,
           y = value,
           group = stat,
           linetype=stat)) +
```

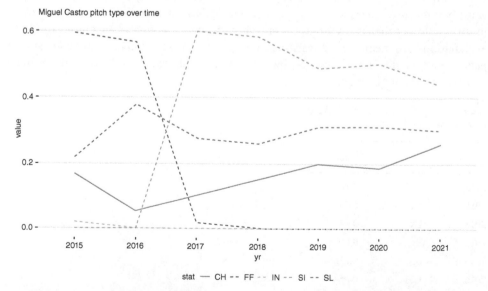

Figure 3.4 Pitch type by year showing the changing pitch type mix contextualizing the ERA change.

```
geom_line(aes(color=stat)) +
ggtitle(chartTitle) + theme_hc()
```

Once again to create the dynamic JavaScript plot, the year column needs to be reclassified as a factor type. This is declared with `as.factor` applied to the `yr` column. The `echarts4r` package will change its behavior when presented with a grouped "tibble" data object. The `dplyr` function `group_by` accepts a data frame and grouping column name and then returns the grouped "tibble" object. As part of the "tidy-verse," the author prefers the pipe forward operation and column names can be passed without quotes. The grouped data is forwarded to the base e-charts layer `e_charts` which needs the *y*-axis column name, `yr`. The next layer is the declaration of a line chart referencing the `value` column. Additional JavaScript functionality is added so that users can download a static version of the image with `e_toolbox_feature`. The last three layers refer to the aesthetics, the functionality of a mouse over tooltip, and chart title referring to the `chartTitle` object, respectively. Although line type is not adjusted by pitch type, a user can mouse over to get specific information and a different theme would change line colors automatically. Here, gray was chosen for publication but is easily adjusted. Figure 3.5 is a recreation of the preceding line chart but with added interactive functionality when presented in a web browser.

```
pitchPropsLong$yr <- as.factor(pitchPropsLong$yr)
pitchPropsLong %>% group_by(stat) %>%
  e_chart(yr) %>%
  e_line(value) %>%
  e_toolbox_feature(feature = "saveAsImage") %>%
  e_theme('gray') %>%
  e_tooltip() %>%
  e_title(chartTitle)
```

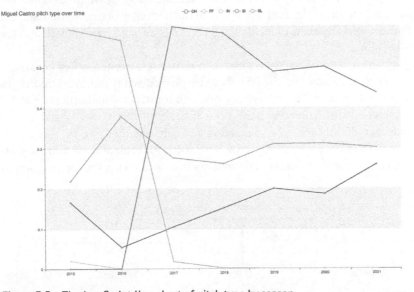

Figure 3.5 The JavaScript line chart of pitch type by season.

Another contributing factor to the pitcher's ERA change may be mechanic adjustments resulting in different speeds even within the same pitch types. In this example, the player has over 5000 individual pitches which need to be summarized. One method for exploring this is tabular with the `group_by` function. In the following code, the individual pitch data is passed to dplyr's functions `group_by` and then `summarize`. The intent is to first group by a column of factors, representing seasons, and then for each grouping apply summarizing function from base-R. Therefore, `summarize` needs declared column names along with the functionality to be applied. In succession the `mean`, `min`, and `max` are applied to the `MPH` column. Remember to separate these summarizations by commas. The result is a "tibble" data table with five columns: the "year," "Pitch" type, "mean," "min," and "max." As expected, this table will have the average, minimum, and maximum miles per hour at release *for each season and pitch type*. For example, in the 2015 season, pitch type "SL" had an average release velocity if 83.3 MPH (134 KPH) while 2020 "SL" averaged 86.6 MPH (139 KPH). This can be observed by applying `head` and then `tail` on the objects to review the first and last six rows of the summarized data.

```
mphStats <- pitchStats %>%
  group_by(year, Pitch) %>%
  summarize(mean = mean(MPH),
            min = min(MPH),
            max = max(MPH))
head(mphStats)
tail(mphStats)
```

Another method for exploring the velocity data is with a box and whisker plot. In a box plot, the inner two quartiles, representing 50% of the data, are illustrated as the "box." The heavier line in the middle represents the median of the distribution. The "whiskers" extend outward from the box accounting for the final quartiles. Additionally the dots to the left and right of the whiskers representing individual outlier values in the distribution. Overall, these components let the audience estimate the normalcy of the distribution, the number of outliers, and any skew of the data. Figure 3.6 is a visual representation to the box and whisker plot.

Returning to the `pitchStats` data, some manipulation is needed before constructing the box plots. Specifically, the data needs to be pivoted with `pivot_longer` as before. The intent is to review the pitch type by year and construct visual using the `MPH` statistic distribution. Thus, `pivtot_longer` will accept `Pitch`, `MPH`, and `year` from the `pitchStats` data frame. The interacting key columns are `Pitch` along with `year`. Therefore, the key-value pairing is the `MPH` value for each of these two interacting keys. The column names are simply `stat` and `value`. Reviewing the `boxes` output

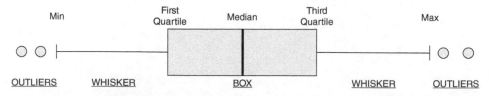

Figure 3.6 A basic explanation of a box plot illustrating a distribution.

in console may aid in understanding this data manipulation step which did *not* change any values themselves.

```
boxes <- pivot_longer(data = pitchStats[,c('Pitch', 'MPH',
'year')],
                cols = -c(year, Pitch),
                names_to = "stat",
                values_to = "value")
```

As observed in Figure 3.3, the ERA started to climb in 2017. Further, in Figure 3.4, the "FF" pitch type decreased suddenly in 2017 and was not identified in any statistics thereafter. As a result, the following code subsets the long form data from 2017 to 2021 and when the `Pitch` variable is not equal to "FF." The exclamation operator is a "negation." This means it negates the proceeding equals sign in the code below. Thus the two, `!=` need to be next to each other for the `subset` to perform as expected. The second line merely changes the `year` variable from numeric to factor so that `ggplot` can order the box plots correctly.

```
boxes <- subset(boxes, boxes$year>=2017 & boxes$Pitch !='FF')
boxes$year <- as.factor(boxes$year)
```

Before constructing the plot, the following code dynamically updates the chart title in an object `chartTitle`. Once again, the `paste` command is employed referring to the pre-existing `playerFirst` and `playerLast` objects with a contextualizing string.

```
chartTitle <- paste(playerFirst, playerLast, "pitch MPH over
time")
```

Finally, constructing the box plots is straightforward with the `facet_grid` layer. To begin, call `ggplot` with the long form data object, `boxes`. The x-axis will be the `year` factor column while the y-axis is declared as the `value` column. Obviously, the data needs to be grouped by year when reviewing the distributions, thus the `group` aesthetics is again declared as the `year` column. The next layer, `geom_boxplot`, declares the box plots themselves. At this point the pitch type is not incorporated in the visual. The important layer giving context to the pitch type is the `facet_grid` layer. This command forms a plot matrix defined by rows and the column variable then populates the visuals into each section of the plot matrix. Here, the x–y axes remain the same for all `Pitch` types but each pitch's corresponding box plot is separated as a column of visuals. This makes discrete comparisons easier for the audience. The last three layers, `theme_hc`, `theme` with `legend.position = "none"`, and the `ggtitle`, represent final aesthetics for the plot. Overall, it is a best practice to remove visual clutter like legends with faceted visualizations. Figure 3.7 is the resulting plot of box and whiskers by year and pitch type for easy comparison.

```
ggplot(boxes, aes(x=year, y=value, group = year)) +
geom_boxplot(aes(fill=value)) +
facet_grid(Pitch ~ .) +
theme_hc() +
theme(legend.position = 'none') +
ggtitle(chartTitle)
```

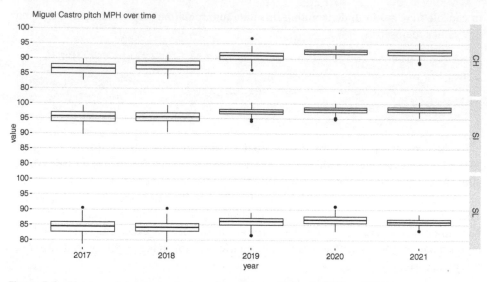

Figure 3.7 The box plots demonstrate an increasing velocity for "CH" and "SI" in particular.

Reviewing the visual along with the `mphStats` data object, there is a clear trend among the most frequent pitch types. This is evident in the "CH" type because the median value in 2017 is slightly above the 85-MPH line. By 2020, the corresponding "CH" median line is clearly above the 90-MPH line. For a more explicit comparison, the "CH" pitch type is subset below. Not only does the box plot show the increasing overall distribution, but this subset shown in Table 3.6 illustrates that the maximum 2017 velocity is 89.6 MPH but by 2020, the player's minimum pitch speed is higher at 89.8 MPH! Perhaps the player's changing pitch types while simultaneously and consistently increasing their speed have led to deteriorating accuracy resulting in the increased ERA.

```
CHtype <- subset(mphStats, mphStats$year>=2017&
mphStats$Pitch=="CH")
```

To recreate a facet wrap with `echarts4r` is more complicated, with more data manipulation and then requiring a either a custom function or repeatedly building plots in a loop. First, the original `pitchStats` data frame is reduced to only `Pitch`, `MPH`, and `year`. Next, the `boxPlotDF` data frame is reduced to only rows containing the

Table 3.6 Showing the maximum value in 2017 being surpassed as the minimum speed by 2020.

Year	Pitch	Mean	Min	Max
2017	CH	86.2	82.4	89.6
2018	CH	87.6	82.8	91
2019	CH	90.6	85.9	96.7
2020	CH	92.3	89.8	94.5
2021	CH	92.0	87.5	95.3

"CH," "SI," and "SL" pitch types. This is done with `grepl`. The `grepl` function is a global regular expression pattern match returning a logical outcome. Essentially, if a pattern is found one or more times in a text vector, the function will return TRUE, otherwise FALSE. Since it employs regular expressions, multiple patterns can be matched with the `|` operator. This "pipe" operator is an OR operator between character strings. In this code, the three pitch types are separated by the `|` so that "CH" OR "SI," OR "SL" are returned. The third code section orders the data frame by two variables. First the data frame is ordered by the `year` variable; then within a year, the `Pitch` is ordered from slowest pitch to fastest. In order for the chart to be ordered correctly, the `Pitch` column is declared as a factor. Lastly, another `subset` is employed to reduce the number of plots for a more visually appealing output. Here, only years between 2017 and 2020 are kept.

```
boxPlotDF <- pitchStats[,c('Pitch', 'MPH', 'year')]
boxPlotDF <- boxPlotDF[grepl('CH|SI|SL', boxPlotDF$Pitch),]
boxPlotDF <- boxPlotDF[ with(boxPlotDF, order(year, Pitch)),]
boxPlotDF$Pitch <- as.factor(boxPlotDF$Pitch)
boxPlotDF <- subset(boxPlotDF,
                    boxPlotDF$year>=2017 &
                    boxPlotDF$year<=2020)
```

Now that the data has been adjusted, a loop to construct the plots within a list object is needed. In case the code is used with other grouping or statistics variables, some convenience objects are declared as `grp` and `stat` objects, respectively. Next, `allPlots` is an empty list object which will be declared iteratively within the for loop.

```
grp <- 'Pitch'
stat <- 'MPH'
allPlots <- list()
```

The loop will repeat once for each year. This is dynamically declared by calculating the `unique` values in the `year` column. This is nested within the `length` function to capture the total number of unique years in the player's statistics data frame. The code setting up the loop is functionally equivalent to `1:4` but is dynamic so that it will function regardless of a player's respective tenure. The first operation in the loop is to create a temporary data frame object `df` using subset. The `df` object is the pitch data for a single year. Next, this is passed to the `dplyr` function `group_by_` with a trailing underscore, to accept a variable which will be replaced by the `grp` object. As is standard for `echarts` the `%>%` forwarding operator will pass objects when building plot layers. The grouped object is forwarded to the basic `e_charts` layer to instantiate a visual. The next layer declares a box plot with `e_boxplot_` command. Similar to the `group_by_` function there is a trailing underscore. In both cases, this denotes referring to an object rather than a column name. Here, `stat` is passed along with a parameter to remove the outlier dots from the boxplots. As has been shown elsewhere, the `e_toolbox_feature` adds the ability to statically save the plot followed by `e_theme` prebuilt aesthetics and finally a `e_tooltip` so used can get specific information during mouse-overs. Once again a chart title is dynamically created within `e_title` by employing the `paste` function with `playerFirst` and `playerLast`. The last parameter of the title character utilizes the `unique` function applied to the `year` column coupled with the loop's `i` variable. This means the year within the title automatically changes with each completion of the loop as `i` iterates from `1` to `4` in this example. After the title is declared another layer is added so that `e_charts4r` will recognize that the multiple plots are part of the same group.

The `e_group` function needs a unique denoting the plots within a particular group. This parameter is called "chartGrp" but could be any string name for the group. This will be explained further in the code after the loop. The next player adds a user interface to zoom the data, changing the *y*-axis. The `e_datazoom` function requires the axis to be assigned to which is `y_index=0` followed by the type of user input which is the `slider`. This is completed by preemptively zooming the values to between `75` MPH and `100` MPH.

Lastly, the list object `allPlots` element is declared so that the first `i` corresponds to the first loop `eChart` plot, and so on.

```
grp <- 'Pitch'
stat <- 'MPH'
allPlots <- list()
for(i in 1:length(unique(boxPlotDF$year))){
    df <- subset(boxPlotDF, boxPlotDF$year==unique(boxPlotDF$y
    ear)[i])
    eChart <- df %>%
      group_by_(grp) %>%
      e_chart() %>%
      e_boxplot_(stat, outlier = F)%>%
      e_toolbox_feature(feature = "saveAsImage") %>%
      e_theme('gray') %>%
      e_tooltip() %>%
      e_title(paste(playerFirst,
                    playerLast,
                    stat,
                    unique(boxPlotDF$year)[i])) %>%
      e_group("chartGrp") %>%
      e_datazoom(y_index = 0, type = "slider", start = 75, end
      = 100)
    allPlots[[i]] <- eChart
}
```

Although this is done with a loop, another option is to construct customized function that would accept the data frame and parameters. While for loops may be slower and considered less robust code, loops are more readily understood for the novice programmer.

Before the plots can be rendered, the plots should be programmatically connected. This will allow the user to zoom in on one chart and the other charts will adjust exactly to the same zoom level rather than having four independent sliders. Additionally, as a user mouse-overs a chart, the tooltip for all charts for the same pitch type will appear. To connect the plots, declare the last plot as connected to all other plots in the list with `e_connect_group` along with the string group name. Admittedly this code may not be intuitive but has the effect that the fourth slider is recognized with all other visuals in the list along with connected tooltips, thereby improving the user interface among all plots.

```
allPlots[[length(allPlots)]] <- allPlots[[length(allPlots)]] %>%
e_connect_group("chartGrp")
```

Finally, to facet multiple `e_charts` in a single view use the `e_arrange` function. This function accepts any number of e chart plot objects. It requires the layout declared as integers for `rows` and `columns`. In this example, one row and four columns are declared so that all four plots in the list are aligned on a single row. Depending on the number of plots, the row and column inputs should be adjusted. Figure 3.8 is a screenshot demonstrating the four dynamic plots with a mouse-over for a single pitch type.

```
e_arrange(allPlots[[1]],
allPlots[[2]],
allPlots[[3]],
allPlots[[4]],
rows = 1, cols = 4)
```

At the time of writing, the `CalledStrike` package is under active development. The package provides function for graphing baseball Statcast data. The Statcast system is a series of tracking devices used in every major league baseball ballpark to automatically account for high-speed, high-accuracy player abilities. Instead of web scraping as was shown previously, the `collect_player` function downloads it directly for a single player and season. This information is from a "mirror" repository of the official data rather than the official tracking service. Here, the code is downloading Miguel Castro's 2020 pitching data for the 2020 season. Once again, the name parameter is constructed dynamically to decrease the number of places to edit in the script, but the input could be declared as a string explicitly instead.

```
player <- collect_player(paste(playerFirst, playerLast),
Season = 2020, Batter = F)
```

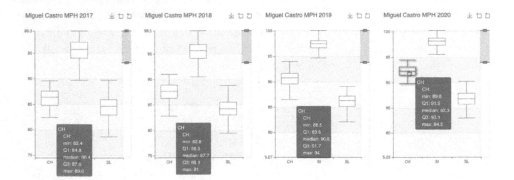

Figure 3.8 A screenshot of the JavaScript box plots for pitch type by year according to MPH.

The package convenience function for constructing a heatmap of pitch location is simply `location_compare`. This function accepts the single season pitch location data from `player`.

```
location_compare(player)
```

However, this function does not create a pitch location by type when accepting the entire data frame. It can be accomplished with additional data manipulation, but it is easier to employ `ggplot`'s `facet_wrap` rather than changing the underlying data structure. For a similar pitch location heatmap, first create a base layer with the `player` data frame and the *x*-axis declared with column `plate_x` and *y*-axis as column `plate_z`. Although one may expect this to be `plate_y`, it is the *z*-coordinate that represents the position when the ball passes over the front of home plate. To construct a heatmap employs the `geom_density_2d` layer. This function needs a `contour_var` parameter. In this case, the string `ndensity` scales the visual to a maximum of 1. This differs from the other input option `count` representing the number of pitches per group or a raw count. Scaling ensures the proportionality is understood proportionally rather than being impacted by raw numbers in case the player has a seldom used pitch type. The `CalledStrike` library provides a `ggplot` layer which adds a prebuilt strike zone in red. To do so, add the `add_zone` layer. The *x* and *y* axes need to be scaled so that the strike zone is placed in the center of the visual for proper interpretation. The `xlim` and `ylim` layers provide the proper axis scaling limited.

```
pitchLocs <- ggplot(player, aes(plate_x, plate_z)) +
  geom_density_2d_filled(contour_var = "ndensity") +
  add_zone() +
  xlim(-2.5, 2.5) +
  ylim(0, 5)
pitchLocs
```

At this point, `pitchLocs` represents all pitches similar to the `location_compare`. Next, clean up the overall aesthetics and apply the facet. This is done by adding a prebuilt theme, `theme_hc`. Then, the standard `theme` layer removes the legend and axes' titles. The `ggtitle` dynamically declares the overall plot title again. Next, the aspect ratio of all visuals will be fixes with `coord_equal`. A scaled coordinate system forces a ratio between the physical data representation data onto the axes. Finally, the `facet_wrap` is added along with the faceting variable name `pitch_name` by all *x–y* values. Figure 3.9 represents the faceted 2020 player pitch heatmap.

```
pitchLocs + theme_hc() +
  theme(legend.position = "none",
        axis.title.x = element_blank(),
        axis.title.y = element_blank()) +
  ggtitle(paste(playerFirst, playerLast, 'Pitch Location')) +
  coord_equal() +
  facet_wrap(pitch_name ~ .)
```

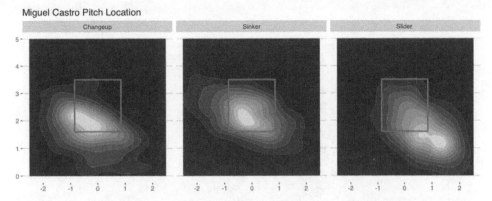

Figure 3.9 The pitch location heatmaps demonstrate the player's preference for sliders to be in a different location compared to both sinkers and changeups.

In addition to `echarts4r` another useful JavaScript visual package is `rbokeh`. This is a port of python's "Bokeh" package from Anaconda. The package provides interactive web-based modern visualizations and has been optimized even for plots with a lot of data points. Similar to `echarts4r` this package utilizes the `%>%` as shown below. First, forward the `player` data frame to the bokeh `figure` layer to instantiate a plot. The plot has a declared aspect ratio of 300 by 300 in pixels but can be adjusted for improved aesthetics. The `ly_crect` layer adds a centered rectangle to the figure at the specified coordinates. This rectangle is made semitransparent with the `alpha` parameter but in actuality represents the strike zone. The last layer is `ly_hexbin`. While not a heatmap, a hexbin plot is similar. This plot type groups multiple data points into a single hexagon shape. The color of each hexagon represents the number of points inside the bin. The `ly_hexbin` needs the *x* and *y* column names and the `alpha` parameter is adjusted to the strike zone rectangle is more easily perceived. Within this layer, `xbins` is changed to improve the output. Similar to bins in a histogram, this tuning parameter will affect the overall bins and therefore audience interpretation of the distribution. Figure 3.10 is a hexbin JavaScript plot for all pitches in the data set. The benefit of a hexbin plot that is interactive is that the specific count within each bin can be obtained with a mouse tooltip.

```
player %>%
figure(width = 300, height = 300) %>%
  ly_crect(0, 2.5,
           width = 2,
           height = 2,
           color = 'red',
           alpha = 0.5) %>%
  ly_hexbin(plate_x,
            plate_z,
            xbins = 15,
            alpha = 0.7)
```

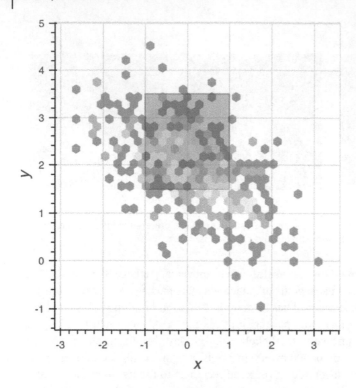

Figure 3.10 Miguel Castro's 2020 pitch locations as shown with hexbins.

Facet wrapping with `rbokeh` is possible with a list and custom function. The function will iterate over each list element to construct the multiple plots. The list is then placed in a special plot grid function from `rbokeh`. To begin, let's `split` the entire data frame by the factor column `pitch_name`. The resulting object is a "ragged" list. This means the subset data frames will each have a different number of rows.

```
pitchLst <- split(player, player$pitch_name)
```

Next, apply the `lapply` function to the `split` list. `lapply` accepts a list and a function to iterate on each list element. Often this can be a standard function from base-R or a package. However, in this code an unnamed function is declared with `function` and a single input `x`. The `x` input is the first element, a data frame of a single pitch type. After completing the function, the `lapply` command will reapply the custom function so that `x` is applied to the second list element, and so on. For the most part, the customized function behaves similar to the previous single plot. There are two differences within the `ly_hexbin` layer. Specifically, the parameter `data` is declared as `x` so that the data is explicitly declared for each input to the custom function. Additionally, the `xbins` input is reduced to 10. This is because the raw count is naturally smaller for these subsections of the overall data now that the data has been `split`.

```
figs <- lapply(pitchLst, function(x) {
  figure(width = 300, height = 300) %>%
    ly_crect(0, 2.5,
             width = 2,
```

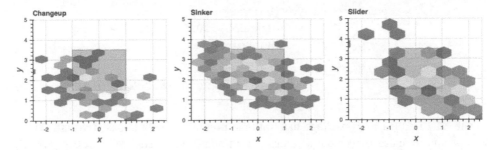

Figure 3.11   The faceted hexbin with JavaScript user tooltips.

```
            height = 2,
            color = 'red',
            alpha = 0.5) %>%
 ly_hexbin(plate_x,
           plate_z,
           data = x,
           xbins = 10,
           alpha = 0.7)})
```

Lastly, the `figs` is a list object where elements are JavaScript plot objects. This list is passed to `grid_plot`. Rather than a true facet from a single column in a single data frame, this command will create a grid and place each list element plot into it. In theory these can be unique and from different data sources though this is not the case in this example. In the end the effect of the grid plot is similar to the facet wrap observed with static `ggplot` images. The inputs to `grid_plot` explicitly declare each visual's coordinates, thereby ensuring proper alignment. The resulting faceted `rbokeh` plot is represented in Figure 3.11.

```
grid_plot(figs,
          xlim = c(-2.5, 2.5),
          ylim = c(0,5))
```

Examining a Single Batter Analytically

Switching to offense, similar statistical tracking information can aid batters. First, let's declare a single player as a variable. Christian Yelich is a left-handed batter. In the 2019 season, his average was 0.329 which means he was getting a hit nearly in one out of three at bats. In the 2020 season, the player's average slumped to 0.205. In that season hits were closer to one in five.

```
batter <- "Christian Yelich"
```

Collecting at bat data for this player is straight forward with `collect_player` from the `CalledStrike` namespace. Given the significant drop off in performance season to season, the function will be applied twice to collect both seasons for visual comparison.

```
batterYrA <- collect_player(batter,
                             Season = 2019, #.329 batting average
                             Batter = T)

batterYrB <- collect_player(batter,
                             Season = 2020, #.205 batting average
                             Batter = T)
```

The `CalledStrike` package has multiple prebuilt `ggplot`-based visuals which accept one or more player data frames. To automatically visualize a `facet_wrap`, simply pass in a list of player data frames to the numerous package visual functions. For example, to obtain a heatmap of the probability of a batter swing by location by year, the list is passed into the `swing_plot` function. It is evident the probability of player swing changed location between the seasons in Figure 3.12. In "Group 1" representing the productive 2019 season, the player swing probability was evenly distributed within the strike zone. In contrast, in "Group 2," the less successful 202 season, the probability of a swing is less diffuse, and actually upon close inspection, the high probability location extends vertically outside the strike zone. The player was demonstrating less discipline, chasing pitches that were high while also limiting their location width.

```
df <- list(batterYrA, batterYrB)
swing_plot(df)
```

The following code examines the actual hits not just probability of a swing. To manually build a faceted `ggplot`, the data frames need to be combined and a grouping variable declared. The `rbind` command will row bind two data frames as long as the columns are shared. The `year` command from `lubridate` will extract the year from a `Date` class vector. In this code, a new column `yr` is defined on the left side of the assignment operator while the `year` command is applied to the `game_date` vector.

```
bothYrs     <- rbind(batterYrA, batterYrB)
bothYrs$yr <- year(bothYrs$game_date)
```

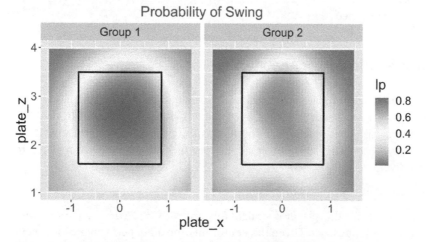

Figure 3.12 The year-over-year change in swing probability for the batter.

The `hit_location` column contains zone information when a hit occurs and NA if no hit is recorded. Thus, the `subset` command is applied to filter the data. The logical condition employs `is.na` and checks then the return value is equal to TRUE. `is.na` indicates if an element is missing or NA within a vector and returns a Boolean TRUE or FALSE.

```
onlyHits <- subset(bothYrs,
                   is.na(bothYrs$hit_location)==F)
```

Now that the data has been subset, a `ggplot` can be instantiated with *x* and *y* axes declared as `plate_x` and `plate_z`, respectively. The two-dimensional kernel density plot layer is added with `geom_density_2d_filled`. Anther strike zone is added with `add_zone`. One can declare a `Color` parameter as a string but the default is "red" as shown. Similar to previously done, the `xlim` and `ylim` coordinate values are declared. Then, the `facet_wrap` declaration splits the plots by `yr`. There are other interesting facet variables in the data set such as changing `yr` to `pitch_name`. Once again, the `ggtitle` layer dynamically adds an appropriate plot title using the `paste` function. The legend is removed within the `theme` layer and the overall aesthetics are set to High Charts with `theme_hc`. Figure 3.13 shows that between years, the sources of hits were dramatically different. In 2019, the batter was able to make contact in the upper right of the strike zone while not as much in 2020. This particular batter stands on the first base side to the right of home plate. Thus in 2019 the batter had success with hits up and inside of the strike zone while in 2020 this productivity diminished for actual hits. This is evident within the dense most contours of Figure 3.13.

```
ggplot(onlyHits,aes(x=plate_x,y=plate_z)) +
  geom_density_2d_filled() +
  add_zone(Color = 'red') +
```

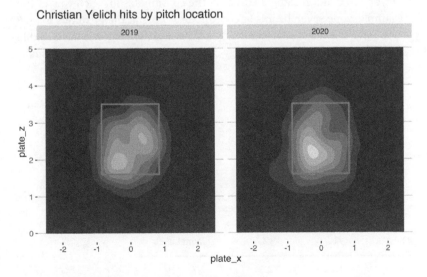

Figure 3.13 The different hit locations by season.

```
xlim(-2.5, 2.5) +
ylim(0, 5) +
facet_wrap(yr ~.) + #pitch_name
ggtitle(paste(batter,'hits by pitch location')) +
theme_hc() +
theme(legend.position = 'none')
```

A more traditional baseball pitch view is by predetermined zones numbered one to nine. Any pitch passing the plate in the geographic location for a zone is assigned a factor level representing a grouping rather than an explicit singular location. The following code sets up the basic strike zone areas as a data frame. These represent the coordinates that `ggplot` will later refer to when constructing a zone-based visual. This is why the columns are a series of x–y pairs.

```
strikeZones <- data.frame(
  x1         = rep(-1.5:0.5, each = 3),
  x2         = rep(-0.5:1.5, each = 3),
  y1         = rep(1.5:3.5, 3),
  y2         = rep(2.5:4.5, 3),
  #z = factor(c(.13, .13, .01, .15, .05, .27, .11, .07, .07))
  zoneLabel = factor(c(7, 4, 1,
8, 5, 2,
9, 6, 3)))
```

The following `ggplot` code will help understand the layout of the strike subzones without regard to a specific batter. It begins by creating the plot referring to the `strikeZones` data frame and then defining the x–y axes' limits similar to previous visuals. Both `xlab` and `ylab` are set to an empty string which has the effect of removing the labels altogether. Next `geom_rect` adds the actual zones as rectangles of the overall strike zone. This layer will add a rectangle based on the coordinates for each row of the data frame. For example, zone seven begins at coordinates –1.5 and then extends to –0.5 along the x-axis. Similarly, the y-axis coordinates start at 2.5 and then extends to 1.5. Table 3.7 is a portion of the `strikeZone` data for easy comparison in the subsequent visual.

```
subZones <- ggplot(data = strikeZones) +
  xlim(-2.5, 2.5) + xlab("") +
  ylim(0, 5) + ylab("") +
  geom_rect(aes(xmin = x1, xmax = x2,
                ymin = y2, ymax = y1, fill = zoneLabel),
            color = "grey20")
```

Table 3.7 The x–y coordinates for two strike subzones.

x1	x2	y1	y2	zoneLabel
–1.5	–0.5	1.5	2.5	7
–1.5	–0.5	2.5	3.5	4

The next layer adds labels with `geom_text`. The zone labels are defined using the `zoneLabel` column. The coordinates are adjusted so that the text label is centered exactly halfway between the corresponding x and y coordinates. This ensures the label is placed centrally for each rectangle. Specifically, the equation for both x and y `x1 + (x2 - x1)/2` will calculate the central point along each axis. The last two will simplify the visual to black and white with `theme_bw` while also removing the legend within the `theme` layer. Running the next code chunk now will simply add labels 1–9 for each subzone.

```
subZones +
  geom_text(aes(x = x1 + (x2 - x1)/2,
                y = y1 + (y2 - y1)/2, label = zoneLabel),
            size = 7, fontface = 2, color = I("grey20")) +
  theme_bw() +
  theme(legend.position = "none")
```

Before running the code to construct the visual, let's understand the proportionality of the batter's hits by zones by year. First, create `hitTally` with `table` applied to the `hit_location` variable of `onlyHits` interacting by the `yr` column. There are definitely other methods to tally data within the tidy-verse but this function is from base-R making it likely to remain unchanged. `hitTally` is a tally of the zone among all hits by year. Next, apply `prop.table` which calculates proportions by column. This is specified with the `2` parameter and would be `1` if proportions were calculated by rows. Often floating-point numbers are not useful for visuals because it adds visual clutter. The `round` function will accept the default eight-digit decimal proportions and adjust them to a specified number of places. The result of this effort is demonstrated in Table 3.8.

```
hitTally <- table(onlyHits$hit_location)
hitTally <- proportions(hitTally)
hitTally <- round(hitTally, 3)
```

Table 3.8 The player's proportion of hits for both seasons.

	2019	2020
1	0.038	0.03
2	0.266	0.406
3	0.072	0.086
4	0.125	0.117
5	0.049	0.051
6	0.067	0.046
7	0.125	0.122
8	0.145	0.086
9	0.112	0.056

Finally, let's pivot this data longer and reapply within the zone visual. To do so, simply call `as.data.frame` on the table object. When coercing the table object class `as.data.frame` will "stack" the data into a triple with the first column as zones, the second as the season and a `Freq` column representing the season's proportion. To ensure the data is understood, the column `names` are declared explicitly using `c` and corresponding strings. It is important because the third column is not a "frequency" as the automated name may imply. Instead, it is a proportionality.

```
hitTally <- as.data.frame(hitTally)
names(hitTally) <- c('zoneLabel','yr','proportion')
```

A `left_join` is once again employed to append data. In this code chunk the predefined zone coordinates are joined as the right-hand table to the long form proportional seasonal data as the left table. The effect is that corresponding `x1`, `x2`, `y1`, and `y2` columns are added by specific zone.

```
hitTally <- left_join(hitTally, strikeZones, by = "zoneLabel")
```

The following code is largely the same as the previous `ggplot` visual code. However, the data object has been changed to `hitTally`. Additionally, within the `geom_text` layer, the `label` parameter is adjusted to the `proportion` column. Lastly, a new layer to `facet_wrap` by year is added. The result is a side-by-side nine zone strike zone by year. Figure 3.14 clearly shows that in zone two, the upper row middle zone, the proportion increased significantly. The batter is getting more hits from this region, which may illustrate less plate discipline, certainly a changing batting strategy which according to the seasonal averages resulted in deteriorating performance year to year.

```
ggplot(data = hitTally) +
  xlim(-2.5, 2.5) + xlab("") +
```

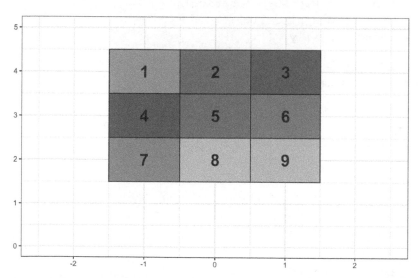

Figure 3.14 The proportion of hits by predefined zone by season showing a changed player behavior.

```
ylim(0, 5) + ylab("") +
geom_rect(aes(xmin = x1, xmax = x2,
              ymin = y2, ymax = y1, fill = zoneLabel),
          color = "grey20") +
geom_text(aes(x = x1 + (x2 - x1)/2,
              y = y1 + (y2 - y1)/2, label = proportion),
          size = 7, fontface = 2, color = I("grey20")) +
theme_bw() +
theme(legend.position = "none") + facet_wrap(yr~.)
```

Extending the Chapter Methods

There are multiple ways to extend the lessons of this chapter. For example, you can create more visuals than those covered here. In fact, the `CalledStrike` library is specifically made with convenience functions for plotting statistical baseball information. In addition to the univariate player analysis and visualizations demonstrated, an interesting aspect of this analysis is the comparative nature of the player-to-player statistics or aggregated to pitching staffs or teams, divisions, or leagues. As is often the case among baseball player personnel, a choice must be made between one or more players to fill a roster. In the past qualitative assessments, observation would have been the primary method for comparison. Now quantitative information and statistical graphs can *supplement* the qualitative expertise of talent scouts. Here is a brief example from the `CalledStrike` package vignette demonstrating the ease of player-to-player assessments for two batters. Keep in mind, you can manually create these charts with `ggplot` and `facet_wrap` for more aesthetic control. Further, the players can easily be switched or the two subsections of data can be changed. For instance, the comparisons of the chart can be before or after an injury or pre or post a trade into a new league. Figure 3.15 shows the comparative chart from one functional call `ls_contour` demonstrating how comparisons can be made easily.

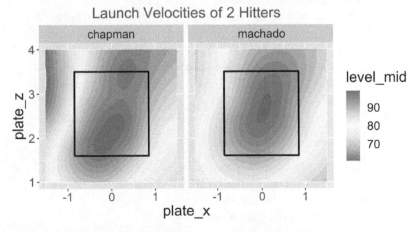

Figure 3.15   The comparison between launch velocities and location among two batters.

```
playerA <- collect_player("Manny Machado",
                          Season = 2019,
                          Batter = T)
playerB <- collect_player("Matt Chapman",
                          Season = 2019,
                          Batter = T)
twoPlayers <- list(machado = playerA,
                   chapman = playerB)
ls_contour(twoPlayers, L = seq(60, 100, by = 2),
           title = "Launch Velocities of 2 Hitters")
```

Exercises

1) Explore the Cleveland Guardians (name changed 2021) player "Shane Bieber" seasonal ERA which is `playerID` `biebesh01`.
   a) Create a line chart of the players ERA statistics for years 2018, 2019, and 2020.

2) Obtain the pitching data for the Cleveland Guardian (name changed in 2021) player "Shane Bieber" for the 2020 season.
   a) Plot the overall pitch location for this player in a single season as a two-dimensional heatmap.
   b) Using `facet_wrap`, reconstruct the heatmap by `pitch_name`.
   c) Using the faceted plot, describe the differenced between the "Changeup," "Slider," and "Knuckle Curve." Are there location similarities or differences among the pitches generally and specifically between these three?

3) Obtain batting data for the Detroit Tigers' player "Harold Castro" for the 2019 and 2020 season.
   a) Arrange the data in a list object.
   b) Plot the probability of a swing as a "heatmap."
   c) Review the plot and summarize the batter's consistency for probability of a swing between the two seasons. Is the player consistent in their approach to batting? Review the player's seasonal batting average, either online or in the existing data. Does the player's consistent probability of a swing translate into a consistent batting average season to season? Performing some online research, review how websites describe the player, that is, is the player a "contact hitter" or "solid line drive hitter" as opposed to a "home run hitter" or "power hitter"?

4) Compare the Cleveland Guardians (name changed in 2021) player "Jake Bauers" and the Los Angeles Angels "Mike Trout" for season 2019.
   a) Obtain their respective data for the season.
   b) Arrange a list object with proper player names.

c) Create a contour plot of exit velocities.

d) Qualitatively describe the batter's difference in this season. Which one has more overall power? Which one shows a larger area for strong hits? Reviewing external seasonal data and online descriptions, which player is considered better more generally (cite the online description supporting this conclusion)?

4

Evaluating Players for the Football Draft

Objectives

- Following the Sample, Explore, Modify, Model and Assess, SEMMA, workflow build various football player statistics models
- Explore the player evaluation data and build dynamic visualizations
- Understand the implications for the annual football player prospect evaluations in terms of being drafted versus not
- Use a KNN binary classification model to classify the probability of being drafted
- Use a KNN multiple classification model to classify the most likely draft round
- Use a KNN regression model to predict the overall pick a player may be selected
- Apply K-means clustering to the player data to identify cohorts by mean values
- Apply K-medoid clustering to the player data to identify cohorts by median values
- Apply an unsupervised, non-Euclidean, algorithm called spherical K-means to separate player prospects and identify the prototypical players within a cluster

R Libraries

vtreat
caret
echarts4r
dplyr
RCurl
ggplot2
ggthemes
tidyr
ggalt
pROC
skmeans

Sports Analytics in Practice with R, First Edition. Ted Kwartler.
© 2022 John Wiley & Sons Ltd. Published 2022 by John Wiley & Sons Ltd.

```
kmed
fst
cluster
data.table
RCurl
```

R Functions

```
data.frame
sum
*
sqrt
/
cosine
getURL
read.csv
sapply
is.na
subset
names
head
summary
table
as.data.frame.matrix
table
rownames
c
rowSums
order
pivot_longer
factor
unique
ggplot
aes
geom_col
theme_hc
ggtitle
e_charts
e_bar
e_tooltip
e_x_axis
```

```
e_toolbox_feature
function
mean
min
max
aggregate
do.call
grep
geom_dumbbell
geom_text
facet_wrap
group_by
summarise
mutate
e_scatter
list
e_flip_coords
ordered
names
designTreatmentsZ
prepare
as.factor
train
plot
predict
confusionMatrix
roc
as.logical
round
nearZeroVar
RMSE
%in%
complete.cases
scale
kmeans
attr
t
apply
pam
skmeans
prop.table
```

Sports Context

In total there are greater than 890 collegiate football teams in the United States. Among them, 130 Division I schools exist. The Division I teams are considered the most competitive and require the most athleticism. Each year the professional American football league evaluates amateur collegiate players, primarily from Division I programs. The goal of the evaluation is to identify top talent for next year's professional season. Given the number of players and the fact that teams are segregated into divisions, apples-to-apples comparisons among players can be difficult. Setting aside the discussion that collegiate sports is not really about amateur athleticism, the Annual Scouting Combine solves the asymmetric evaluation problem by allowing athletes to be measured in specific quantifiable tasks.

The Combine takes place each year at the end of February well after the conclusion of the college football season. In it, over 300 elite athletes perform timed drills in front of team executives, coaches, and other personnel such as medical staff. The four-day event requires concentration by athletes and given their best performance may open up the door to be drafted, resulting in contracts worth millions of dollars and qualitatively fulfilling the childhood dreams of these athletes to play at the highest level. Given the wide-ranging skillsets depending on positions, the athletes are not competing holistically, rather within their defined positions. The primary tangible attribute that the skill evaluations seek to demonstrate is described in Table 4.1. There are other non-tangible attributes such as character and leadership which are generally not considered part of the quantitative assessment of the annual combine.

In order to measure multiple aspects of athleticism, the Combine or "National Invitational Camp" as it is officially named has specific drills. The thinking goes these events, over time, have helped scouts identify talent regardless of the school they went to, the level of competition they faced, the marketing efforts of their agent, or hype generated online or in TV media. To that end the following drills in Table 4.2 have been part of the combine for at least 20 years.

This chapter explores the usefulness of the player level fitness drill data from historical combine events. Since millions of dollars are on the line, football teams are eager to identify the best players and also avoid costly drafting mistakes. Under rules since 2010 teams

Table 4.1 The primary football positions and corresponding attributes measured in the Combine.

Position	Primary tangible evaluation
Quarterback	Arm strength and accuracy
Wide receiver	Agility, body control, strength, quickness, stamina, focus, and hand–eye coordination
Running back	Balance, and vision, stamina to play on many downs
Defensive line and linebacker	Vision, strong arms to fight past defense and tackle
Defensive back	Speed and quickness

Table 4.2 The professional athlete evaluation drills and corresponding justification.

Drill name	Description	Scouting justification
40 Yard dash	Players start in a 3-pt stance and sprint for 40 yards on level ground	Depending on the position, scouts evaluate the acceleration to 10 yards for linemen, the time to travel 10–20 yards for running backs and for wide receivers the time between 20 and 40 yards
Vertical jump	Standing still and flatfooted, players jump as high as they can reaching for the highest flag	This drill evaluates the explosive muscle potential of a player. This can be relevant for wide receivers and defensive safeties who routinely jump for passes
20 Yard shuttle run	Players start in a 3-pt stance begin between two lines spaced 10 yards apart. An athlete must run 5 yards to his right, crouch and touch the line, then run 10 yards touching the opposing line and then sprint back to the starting mid-point	The shuttle run demonstrates lateral movement and the ability to change direction. These skills are especially helpful for evaluating receivers
Bench press	Using 225-pound barbell, players lift the weight from a laying position as many times as possible	The repetitive bench press is a test of strength and stamina. Among other positions, the drill particularly evaluates the strength of a lineman to overpower an opponent
Broad jump	Standing still and flat footed, a player will jump forward landing on both feet and maintaining balance	The distance measured horizontally as opposed to vertically with the vertical drill measures the explosive power in a different set of muscles, namely, the hips. As a result, the broad jump is a good measure of durability and power for running backs
Three-cone drill	Players run a pattern among three cones, touching each one then back to the starting point	This drill helps assess body control, acceleration, and the ability to change direction. This is important among safety, defensive end, and linebacker positions

have an allotted amount allocated to rookie players. On average, the rookie drafted salary is $660,000.[1] This accounts for most teams ~$200 million rookie salary pool divided by the average number of draft picks per team. However, the first overall picks make closer to $40 million in their contract. This means there is less within a team's pool to allocate to later selected athletes in the draft. Thus, having an early round draft pick that does not contribute to the team or worse is waived costs teams a lot of money. Although scouts provide

---

1 Corry, J. (2021, May 7). *Agent's Take: 2021 NFL rookie contract projections for key Round 1 picks, plus a rookie wage scale explainer.* CBSSports.com. https://www.cbssports.com/nfl/news/from-aaron-rodgers-to-deshaun-watson-and-more-predicting-the-outcome-of-nfls-most-pressing-situations.

meaningful qualitative assessments of athleticism and intangible qualities, with so much money on the line, a quantitative approach is justified for agreement both qualitatively and quantitatively.

The data will be sampled, explored, modified, modeled, and assessed following the standard data-modeling SEMMA workflow. The SEMMA workflow is one of standard industry practices useful in organizing an analytical, particularly machine learning, project. This chapter applies quantitative modeling to determine

- The probability an athlete will be drafted in any round.
- An expected draft round for athletes given their Combine drill results which may indicate overrated or underrated expectations.
- Any observed grouping or cluster of athletes which could be understood as elite versus middling or even lower draft expectations.
- Identify the prototypical athlete among each cluster. The center of each cluster, called a centroid, may be the exemplary athlete for that particular group's characteristics. This may mean the "most elite" among top players, the prototypical "average" in another group, and so on.

Technical Context

This chapter utilizes three somewhat related methods. First, the *K*-nearest neighbor (KNN) machine learning algorithm is applied. Although not widely used in today's data science environment, the algorithm is a simple first step to answering two of this chapter objectives mentioned previously. KNN also has the benefit of working with binary and multiclass, even continuous outcomes, so it is a useful elementary tool for novice data scientists. The differences are shown here:

- **Binary classification**—Answers a "Yes/No," "True/False," or "0/1" type problem. The input features like height and weight answer a question with only two possible outcomes.
- **Multi-class classification**—Answers questions with more than two possible outcomes. For example, in business, customers may be classified into the "high-spenders," "mid range spenders," and "unlikely to buy anything." In this scenario, there are three possible outcomes, though in multi-class problems there can be many more possible outcomes states.
- **Continuous regression**—Answers questions where the outcome is along a spectrum of outcomes, for example, building a model to predict the number of points a team will score in a match. There is a minimum and conceivable maximum but overall it is a range of outcomes rather than distinct states like classifications.

In all three methods described above, there is a distinct outcome. In statistics this is called the "dependent variable." The independent variables act as inputs to predict or classify an outcome which depends on these inputs. In machine learning, this relationship is called supervised learning. The KNN algorithm is a supervised modeling approach. This means the algorithm expects an outcome variable, either binary, multi-class, or continuous. The contrast is a family of algorithms under "unsupervised" techniques. These techniques use varying methods to identify different cohorts, known as clusters, within the data according to the patterns observed. Unsupervised learning does not have an outcome variable, such as being drafted or not. In this chapter's player evaluation example, the unsupervised model would attempt to identify two clusters or cohorts of players that may roughly approximate those that have been drafted versus not, for example, by identifying a cluster of faster and stronger players within the evaluation data. Specifically, this chapter employs an unsupervised technique that is less widely known call spherical *K*-means. The spherical *K*-means clustering algorithm employs cosine similarity to identify clusters. This method differs from KNN, in the supervised methods or *K*-means clustering (not covered) in the unsupervised methods because spherical *K*-means does not employ Euclidean distances to identify clusters.

> Supervised learning is a family of algorithms that require an outcome "target" or "dependent" variable. These models predict or classify one column based on the patterns identified in the other informative, input variables.

> Unsupervised learning is a collection of algorithms that seeks to identify clusters or patterns in the data to subset rows into. It does not require an outcome variable.

KNN–Supervised Learning: Binary Classification

KNN stands for *K*-nearest neighbor. The KNN algorithm identifies nearby observations in the training data measured by Euclidean distance. The goal is to classify a new record by reviewing its closeness to the training data observations in a "hyperspace," meaning more than two dimensions. To score a new record, the count of nearby neighbors by each class is performed. The proportion of neighbors from one class or another provides the probability of the new record being one or the other class. There are multiple nuances to this algorithm including scaling the data. To scale data, apply the `scale` function which subtracts the mean average of a column from each value and then divides each value by the standard deviation. Doing so, puts all values on the same scale so one variable does not dominate in the hyperspace distance calculations. Another facet of KNN is the tuning parameter "*K*" which denotes the number of neighbors to include in the tally of class neighbors. Too few may make a model sensitive to the local data structure while too many will default toward the average probability per class. This chapter will use default parameters for employing KNN because traditional machine learning books cover it in greater detail. For now, Figure 4.1 shows how the neighbors determine the new record's likelihood using fictional data with only two variables. In the plot, players C and E were successfully drafted while A, B, and D were not. The new player prospect F is denoted with a question mark. The distance between F and C, F and E, and F and B represents the three closest neighbors. As a result, two of three neighbors were drafted so KNN would assign a 66% (2/3) probability of Player F being drafted.

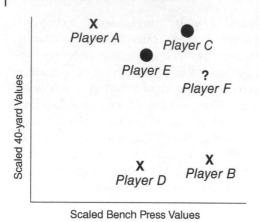

Figure 4.1 Demonstrating KNN with three neighbors and a binary outcome class.

KNN—Supervised Learning: Multi-class Classification

Although this chapter models the simple outcome drafted versus not drafted, the professional football league selects new players in an annual draft according to rounds. First-round draft picks are thought to be more athletic and ready for play versus later round picks. As a result, another way to examine the player data is to create a multi-class model. In this case, the outcome variable has various levels such as "1st round" or "2nd round." Luckily, KNN is one of the few approaches that can be applied to a multi-class problem as well as binary. Coincidentally, KNN can be useful in continuous problems where the outcome variable is not class based but a continuous number. Figure 4.2 has been adjusted with new players and with multiple class levels. Now Player F's closest neighbors include two first-round picks and a second-round pick. KNN would determine that Player F has a 66% chance of being a first-round pick and 33% being chosen in the second. This assumes a *K* value of three.

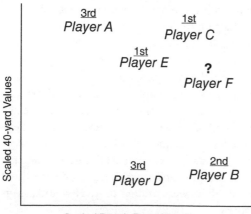

Figure 4.2 Adjusted for multi-class outcomes, player F has a 66% chance of being chosen in the first round of player selection.

Spherical K-means

Rather than a supervised approach with a clear dependent or outcome variable, a clustering approach can also be applied to the data. This "unsupervised" approach will identify cohorts of observations that similar. The practitioner is then left to contextualize the clusters. For example, a cluster of wide receivers with exceptional speed that are drafted in the third round may be identified using an unsupervised method. If the cohorts can be contextualized, the benefits are exploratory and explanatory. On one hand, the contextualization of a cluster may yield interesting insights for the sports management professional. For example, a group of players with particular evaluation results may be an overlooked source of good draft outcomes. This helps elucidate a global phenomenon of the football drafting characteristics. More specifically for new individual draftees, the cluster assignment may explain a specific affiliation to the group that is either contextualized as successful or not. Thus, contextualizing clusters can help understand the whole ecosystem and an individual observation.

There are many clustering techniques. Among the most popular is the *K*-means clustering or *K*-medoid clustering. As expected, each uses the mean or the median, respectively, in the following workflow.

To begin, the number of clusters is declared. For example, three clusters can be defined by the user. Next, a "centroid" or cluster center is randomly placed in the hyperspace of the data, one for each defined cluster. Next, the distance between all points and each centroid is measured. Each point is assigned to the closest centroid. Figure 4.3 shows fictitious observations in a two-dimensional space, with three clusters shown as stars. Illustratively, the distance from each centroid to a point is represented with an arrow. The point central point would be assigned to cluster three because its arrow is the shortest.

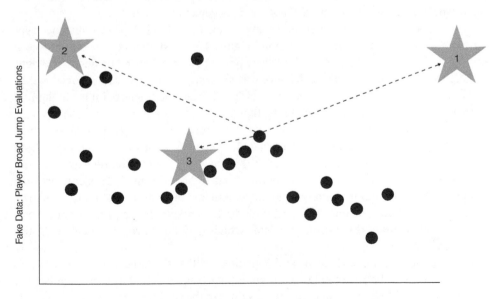

Fake Data: Player Vertical Evaluations

Figure 4.3   Player data with three centroids and distance measures being taken.

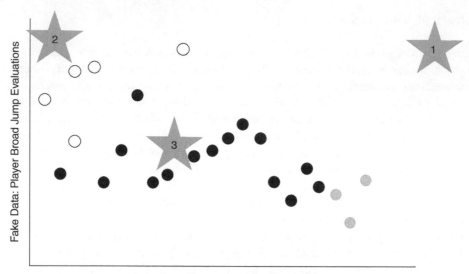

Fake Data: Player Vertical Evaluations

Figure 4.4 The assigned points for each cluster.

When all points are assigned to a cluster, the mean average distance or median average distance between the points and the centroid is calculated. Figure 4.4 has three color-coded points according to the original centroid placement. Notice how cluster one was randomly placed far away but some points were assigned to it. Further, cluster three has points all around but the majority are to the upper right. Lastly, cluster two has some nearby points and two points on the "border" between cluster three.

Regardless of the average measure, the centroid is moved to the average distance spot among the corresponding assigned points. Figure 4.5 shows that cluster one moved a great deal to minimize the distance for its few points. Cluster 3 moved up and to the right a short amount so that its average distance was minimized and cluster two moved within its boundaries but very close to a point was assigned to cluster 3. This point is highlighted with an additional dotted line circle in the figure.

Once the centroids are moved, another distance calculation is performed and once again the points are reassigned to a cluster. In some cases, this means points will be reassigned, such as the one highlighted in Figure 4.5. This process repeats until the centroids are in a place, whereby no points need to be reassigned. This convergence happens after many iterative attempts at movement and reassignment. Figure 4.6 shows a fictitious set of clusters one, two, and three with corresponding points. In the visual, the centroids identify three distinct cluster which may not have been evident in the original visual 4.3.

The difference between *K*-means and *K*-medoids is that the latter is less impacted by outliers. Consider the vector below with an extreme outlier. The mean average is 12.5. This number is not very close to many of the values in the vector-space. The median is 3.5, which is much more representative of the vector space. Thus, if the clustering data has outliers, it is a good practice to use *K*-medoid clustering.

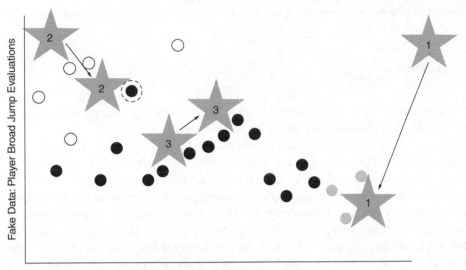

Figure 4.5 The centroids move to minimize either the mean or median distances among assigned points. This causes one point to change affiliation, highlighted by the concentric circle.

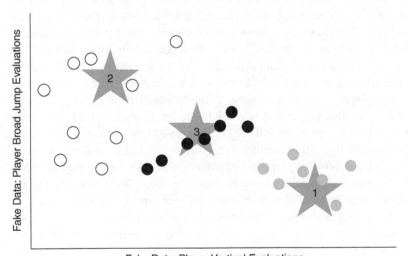

Figure 4.6 The centroids placed where no more points are reassigned and three distinct clusters of points emerge.

- Vector: 1, 2, 3, 4, 5, **60**
  - Mean: 12.5
  - Median: 3.5 (closer to move points in the original vector)

However, both *K*-means and *K*-medoid clustering utilize Euclidean distance. A competing clustering technique is one where the cosine-similarity is used to calculate the distances and then move centroids. The following formula calculates the cosine similarity among points, in this chapter's data, players.

$$\cos(\theta) = \frac{A \cdot B}{\|A\| \|B\|}$$

While the formula may be intimidating, consider the following example with dummy data. Table 4.3 has two attributes among two players.

The numerator of the cosine similarity formula is called the "dot product." To calculate the dot product simply multiple each column by its corresponding value in the other columns, then sum all the operations according to each other column, for example, 65×80 equals 5200. Then, 166×326 equals 54,116. Summing the two arrives at the dot product between player A and player B which is **59,316**. This is repeated for all combinations of columns such as player B to player C which has a dot product of **115,690**.

Moving to the denominator, let's calculate each player combinations' "magnitude." The magnitude is a little more complicated but nonetheless manageable. First, multiple each value by itself, essentially squaring it. For example, 65×65 is 4225 and 166×166 is 27,556. These values are summed to 31,781. Then take the square root of the summed values, here these represent the player's individual height and weight as squared values, but they can be any numeric attribute. The square root of 31781 is **~178.3**. Next, this process is repeated for another column. For player B, 80×80 is 6400, and 326×326 is 106,276. These two values sum to 112,676. Finally, the square root is taken so that the result is **~335.7**. Finally, to obtain the magnitude of player A to player B multiple **~178.3** by **~335.7**. This equals **59,841.09**. If the same process is run on the player B and player C column, the magnitude is **115,690.7**.

Once all dot product and magnitude combinations are calculated, that is, player A to player B, player A to player C, player B to player C, the simple division of dot product by magnitude is calculated. Since player A to player B had a dot product of **59,316** and magnitude of **59,841**, their cosine similarity is **0.9912** (59,316/59,841.09). Similarly, the player B to Player C dot product magnitude combination is 115,690 and **115,690.7**, respectively. Thus, the cosine similarity between player B and player C is **0.9999**. Reviewing the previous table, player A is smaller and would have less similarity than player B or player C. As the cosine similarity approaches 1, the observations are more similar. Another aspect of cosine similarity is that the ratio will always be between 0 (dissimilar) and 1 (identical). The code below shows these calculations as variables using the cosine similarity of two combinations of the `tmp` data frame.

Table 4.3 Illustrative two players' height and weight measurements. Keep in mind these operations are done with more players and measurements.

	Player A	Player B	Player C
Height	65	80	81
Weight	166	326	335

Euclidean Distance   Cosine Similarity

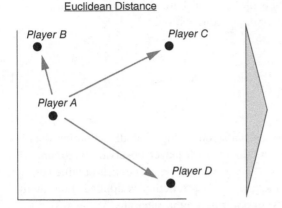
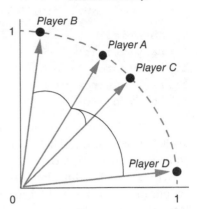

Figure 4.7   The difference between distances measures.

```
tmp <- data.frame(playerA = c(65, 166),
                  playerB = c(80, 326),
                  playerC = c(81, 335))
dotProdAB <- sum(tmp[,1] * tmp[,2])
dotProdBC <- sum(tmp[,2] * tmp[,3])
magnitudeAB <- sqrt(sum((tmp[,1] * tmp[,1]))) *
  sqrt(sum((tmp[,2] * tmp[,2])))
magnitudeBC <- sqrt(sum((tmp[,2] * tmp[,2]))) *
  sqrt(sum((tmp[,3] * tmp[,3])))
dotProdAB / magnitudeAB
dotProdBC / magnitudeBC
```

The latent semantic package has a function that will calculate the cosine similarity matrix from a matrix of values. Using the previous `tmp` example data frame, the following code shows the result which confirms the manual calculations.

```
lsa::cosine(as.matrix(tmp))
```

Figure 4.7 contrasts the difference between Euclidean and cosine distance measures. Euclidean may incorrectly assign player A to its closest counterpart, player B. In contrast, the relative equality between the values of the two vectors would be captured between player A and player C using cosine similarity.

Code—Binary Classification

Let's begin by loading packages for our R environment. First, the variable treatment package, `vtreat`, is used to prepare data frames for modeling rapidly. Next, `caret` supplies functions related to classification and regression training. Throughout this book, visuals are made using various distinct packages. In this chapter, the plots will be dynamic, meaning users can interact with them because they are small web-based JavaScript pages.

R provides many JavaScript visualization options and here the visuals are built with `echarts4r`. Lastly, `dplyr` is loaded for data manipulation.

```
# libraries
library(vtreat)
library(caret)
library(echarts4r)
library(dplyr)
```

After the environment is invoked, the case data containing football evaluation data is loaded. This data is publicly available containing 6,829 player observations among 15 variables. First, the URL is instantiated as `NFLcombineFile`; the data is obtained using `RCurl`'s `getURL` function. Finally, the `read.csv` function is applied. Like many actions in R, there are multiple packages supporting Comma Separated Value, CSV, files. Here, the base `read.csv` is used because the data is small and an optimized function like `fread` from the `data.table` package is not needed.

```
NFLcombineFile <- 'https://raw.githubusercontent.com/
kwartler/Practical_Sports_Analytics/main/C4_Data/combine_
data_2000_2020.csv'
NFLcombineFile <- getURL(NFLcombineFile)
NFLcombine <- read.csv(text = NFLcombineFile)
```

To create a binary classification, the binary outcome of whether or not a player was drafted must be created. In this data, the column `Round` is an integer representing the draft round a player was selected by a professional team. If a player was invited to the evaluation camp but not drafted the `Round` column is `NA`. Adjusting this data to be a binary problem entails identifying any `NA` values in the `Round` column. If a `Round` value is greater than or equal to one the player was drafted, otherwise they were not. Thus, you can accomplish this transformation with an `ifelse` statement but more concisely utilize a negated `sapply` function shown below for the same result. The `sapply` function will apply any function, in this case `is.na` to each element of a vector and return the output as a vector. In this code, `is.na` will result in a TRUE if the value is `NA` and FALSE if not. To switch the returned Boolean values, a leading exclamation point, `!`, is added as a logical operator that switches the `is.na` result. Thus, if a `Round` value is `NA` it is marked as TRUE within `sapply` then switched to FALSE with the exclamation logical operator. The code below adds a column to the data frame called `drafted` because the new column is on the left of the assignment operator.

```
# Make into a binary problem
NFLcombine$drafted <- !sapply(NFLcombine$Round, is.na)
```

This data set is inherently temporal. Drafts by professional teams occur annually. As expected, the column `Year` denotes the year of the evaluation and subsequent draft selection. Contrary to many machine learning modeling workflows, a temporal data set should not be randomly partitioned. It may be that team needs and player attributes evolve over time. This data set should be partitioned using "out of time" sampling. The code below creates a `combineTraining` object for player statistics collected from 2000 to 2016. A validation set is partitioned when the `Year` column is 2017. The remaining years, 2018, 2019, and 2020, represent a holdout set. In all three partitions, the `subset` function is employed. This function subsets when a logical condition is true in the second parameter such as then the `Year` column is less than 2017. Obviously these subsections satisfy the first step in SEMMA sample.

```
combineTraining    <- subset(NFLcombine, NFLcombine$Year<2017)
combineValidation <- subset(NFLcombine, NFLcombine$Year==2017)
combineTest        <- subset(NFLcombine, NFLcombine$Year>=2018)
```

As discussed earlier, the modeling workflow transitions from *sample* to *explore*. It is important to get both tabular data and visual representations of the data during the exploration phase. This is because the human brain is excellent at visual pattern recognition. Let's start with basic column names using `names` and examining the first six rows with `head`.

```
names(combineTraining)
head(combineTraining)
```

From the previous exploration functions there are three possible *y*-variables, `Round`, `Pick`, and the engineered `drafted` columns. To begin, the binary classification model will focus on `drated`. A multi-class classification method could target the `Round` column. Lastly, the `Pick` vector represents a continuous outcome. Regardless of modeling type, be sure to remove the other two *y*-variables otherwise you will invite "target leakage." Leakage is when one *x*-variable uses information that would not be available at the time of prediction. For example, a model would fail if it used the draft round a player was chosen in to predict the "pick" order. This is because at the time the model needs to make the pick prediction, the draft round is not yet known. The two pieces of information are inherently linked. One could prediction stack using a model for the other two variables but that actual `Round` and `drafted` variables represent direct leakage.

Next, another standard practice is to apply the `summary` function and look more closely at the dependent variable `drafted` which was created earlier.

```
summary(combineTraining)
table(combineTraining$drafted)
```

In this data set, the tally of `drafted` is shown in Table 4.4. The table illustrates about 63% of players in the data set are drafted. That is not to say other players do not end up making it to the professional football league. Instead, these undrafted players must find other paths outside of the evaluation combine event. Remember these values are only within the training partition not the validation or holdout sets.

Table 4.4 The result of applying `table` to the `drafted` column.

Drafted = TRUE	Drafted = FALSE
2024	3532

Additional exploratory data analysis is likely needed to become more familiar with the overall tabular data but let's shift our focus to some visualizations with the `ggplot2` and `echarts4r` libraries.

The following code tabulates the player position column by the binary draft status. The `table` function performs the tabulation but returns an R table class. As a result the output is nested in `as.data.frame.matrix` so that table is converted to a data frame. Next, the row name attributes are added back as a column called `Pos`. Since it is now duplicative to have the row names as both object attributes and a column the `rownames` are declared NULL.

```
draftedPos              <- as.data.frame.matrix(
                              table(combineTraining$Pos,
                                  combineTraining$drafted))
draftedPos$Pos          <- rownames(draftedPos)
rownames(draftedPos) <- NULL
```

Another issue of the tabular object result is that the column names are not informative as integers. Instead renaming the columns to `not_drafted`, `drafted`, and `Pos` is more revealing. There are some data inconsistencies with some odd position names like "DB" likely for Defensive Back. These low frequency position oddities often have no draft *or* non-drafted status. As a result, the second line employing `subset` retains all positions that have one or more in either of the first two columns. Lastly, using square brackets and a nested `order` function, the table is sorted. The default parameter for `order` is to sort by the vector as `decreasing=TRUE`. This ordering step does not change the data, only improves the upcoming visual.

```
colnames(draftedPos)s <- c('not_drafted','drafted', 'Pos')
draftedPos              <- subset(draftedPos, rowSums(drafted
Pos[,1:2])>0)
draftedPos              <- draftedPos[order(rowSums(draftedPos
[,1:2])),]
```

To construct a static `ggplot` stacked bar chart, an additional data manipulation step is needed. The `tidyr` function will rearrange the data into a triplet with `pivot_longer`. The data is made to be long, where the `Pos` column is excluded so that the `Pos` and draft status are the key-value pairs. The specific values are recast in a column called `value` and the draft status is renamed as `name`. Next, the position factor ordering is redetermined using `factor` according to this new data orientation. This is inherited into the `ggplot` function call to order the values in increasing order.

```
longDrafted <- pivot_longer(draftedPos, cols = -Pos)
longDrafted$Pos<-factor(longDrafted$Pos, levels =
unique(longDrafted$Pos) )
```

The long format "tidy" data is easily implemented in the `ggplot` call. The aesthetics are declared so that the *x*-axis is the `Pos` column, *y*-axis is the `value` column, and the color fill is defined as the newly created `name` column. The next plot layer is `geom_col`. By default, `geom_col` uses "stat=identity." This means the bar heights are explicit values in the data frame rather than the height being proportional to the number of observations in each group. The premade high charts theme is applied next. The final layer adds the `ggtitle` with a string.

```
ggplot(longDrafted,
       aes(x = Pos, y = value, fill = name)) + geom_col()
  theme_hc() +
  ggtitle('Draft Breakdown by Position')
```

The dynamic D3 equivalent is constructed below. Although not needed, many modern packages use the pipe operator to chain functions. The reasoning behind this is that the code is more easily read compared to traditional R code. The pipe or `%>%` operator merely chains code together in a logical order rather than nesting functions or nonlinear code structures. The pipe operator forwards an object's output to the next function in series. The code below can be described in this manner. Using the original "wide" data `draftedPos` object *then* create a blank `e_charts` visual with the `Pos` column as the *x*-axis *then* add stacked bars with `e_bar` to the chart referring to the `not_drafted` column *then* add to the bar stack again with `e_bar` this time referring to the `drafted` column *then* add a small popup when someone mouses over the chart using `e_tooltip` *then* rotate the *x*-axis labels using `e_x_axis` with the `rotate=45` parameter *then* add a button in the upper right to download the JavaScript visual as a static png file with `e_toolbox_feature` and finally *then* declare a premade color theme `gray` palette. The documentation of `echarts4r` has many premade themes and instructions for declaring your own color palette. While that is a long run on, the statements logically follow the code connected at the `%>%` with each use of the adverb "*then.*" Another nuance of this type of coding is that column names can be declared without quotes as parameters or with the dollar sign. The bar chart in Figure 4.8 is the result of the code.

```
draftedPos %>%
  e_charts(Pos) %>%
```

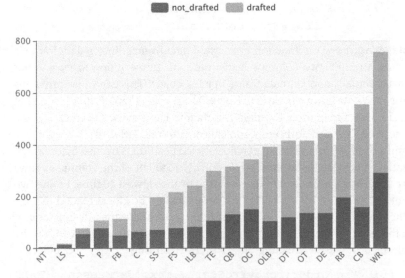

Figure 4.8   A visual comparison of draft to non-draft by position.

```
e_bar(not_drafted, stack = "grp") %>%
e_bar(drafted, stack = "grp") %>% e_tooltip(trigger = "item") %>%
e_x_axis(axisLabel = list(interval = 0, rotate = 45)) %>%
e_toolbox_feature(feature = "saveAsImage") %>% e_theme("gray")
```

One possible takeaway from Figure 4.8 is the larger number of players invited to the event among wide receivers. However, the proportion of drafted corner backs appears to be higher compared to other positions even wide receivers. Thus, high school athletes with aspirations of playing professionally may optimize workouts to be a wide-outs yet may be better served as less exciting defensive cornerbacks.

Let's explore a popular statistic in more detail. The 40-yard dash is a popular metric likely because every fan can run it themselves and compare although the usefulness of the statistic varies among positions. There are many methods to perform the following tasks but this is a simplistic base R way to calculate statistics for the visualization.

First, a custom function is created called `customStats`. The function accepts `x` which is a numeric vector. The function calculates the average, minimum, maximum, and range of values using `mean`, `min`, and `max`, respectively. These summary statistics are combined into a single named vector using the `c` function.

```
customStats <- function(x){
  c(average = mean(x),
    min = min(x),
    max = max(x))
```

Preparing the data for the visualization requires using the `aggregate` function. The goal is to calculate the 40-yard statistics by position *and* the draft status. This is captured in the formula `Fort~Pos+drafted` referring to the column names without quotes. After the formula the data parameter accepts the data frame `combinbeTraining` and finally the `FUN` parameter is declared with `customStats`.

```
fortyYrd <- aggregate(Forty~Pos+drafted,
                      data = combineTraining,
                      FUN = customStats)
```

The output of the `aggregate` function is a nested data frame. Since a data frame is actually a list class, the first two columns begin the data frame followed by another "column" but this is actually another data frame in a list object. This can cause problems so it's best to flatten the data into a simple data frame. Thus, apply the `do.call` function with the `data.frame` function as the first parameter. The second parameter is the nested data frame to be flattened. fortyYrd <- do.call(data.frame, fortyYrd)

Now some simple ordering and removal of a mislabeled position is needed before starting the visualization. The code below employs `order` to the left of the comma so rows within the entire data frame will be ordered decreasing by the slowest 40 time. In line two of the code chunk, a row was labeled as "NT" for nose tackle. The global regular expression pattern matching function, `grep`, will identify this row and return its index number. Once again this is removed with a minus sign on the left side of the comma within the data frame. Table 4.5 is the result of calling `head` on the resulting `fortyYrd` object.

```
fortyYrd <- fortyYrd[order(fortyYrd$Forty.max, decreasing =T),]
fortyYrd <- fortyYrd[-grep('NT', fortyYrd$Pos),]
```

Table 4.5 The summary statistics including average, minimum, maximum, and range by position, draft status.

Pos	Drafted	Forty.average	Forty.min	Forty.max	Forty.diff
OG	FALSE	5.379	4.95	6.05	1.10
OT	TRUE	5.211	4.71	5.99	1.28
OT	FALSE	5.327	4.91	5.85	0.94
C	FALSE	5.251	4.92	5.84	0.92
DT	TRUE	5.075	4.68	5.71	1.03
OG	TRUE	5.257	4.90	5.62	.072

Begin with an empty `ggplot` to create a faceted `ggplot` bar bell plot. Then apply the `ggalt` library function `geom_dumbell`. The data and aesthetics are declared similar to the traditional `geom_segment` with the additional color parameters for the segment end points, here declared as `darkred`. The next two layers add the specific minimum and maximum labels to each of the points. Specifically, `geom_text` coordinates are declared as `Forty.min` and `Pos` variables for the *x*–*y* axes, respectively. The `label` input adds the visual text to the points. The last parameters `color` and vertical adjustments, `vjust`, are merely aesthetic. This layer is essentially repeated so the `Forty.max` coordinates and corresponding labels are added. The `facet_wrap` layer will build two separate but aligned visuals according to the number of levels in the `drafted` column. This layout will make easy comparisons among positions when draft status is TRUE or FALSE. Lastly, the theme is added along with an appropriate title. Figure 4.9 is the result of the faceted 40-yard dash drills by position and draft status. After careful examination, there appear to be some interesting aspects of the data. For example, a WR that runs under 4.34 s will be drafted. This is because the minimum undrafted value is 4.34. A similar relationship occurs for all other positions but the minimum differences are less in other positions requiring less speed such as kickers. Similarly in many positions the maximum 40-yard time for undrafted athletes is higher than the maximum among drafted players. This indicates a hard ceiling for this statistic regardless of the athlete's other evaluations. For example, for wide receivers, no player has been drafted running more than 4.79 s. In comparison the maximum among undrafted is 4.85. This is less pronounced among Tight Ends but is still present in many other positions.

```
ggplot() +
  geom_dumbbell(data=fortyYrd, aes(y=Pos, x=Forty.min,
xend=Forty.max),
               colour_x = 'darkred',
               colour_xend = 'darkred') +
  geom_text(data = fortyYrd,
           aes(x = Forty.min, y = Pos, label = Forty.min),
           color = 'black',
           size = 2,
           vjust = -0.5) +
```

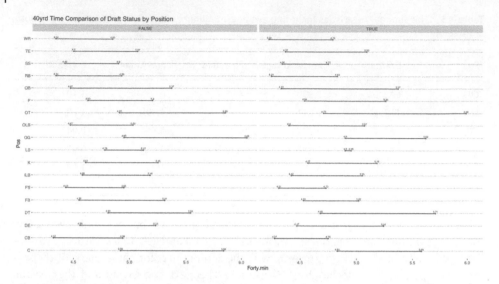

Figure 4.9 This visual compares 40yrd times by position among drafted and undrafted players.

```
geom_text(data = fortyYrd,
          aes(x = Forty.max, y = Pos, label = Forty.max),
          color = 'black',
          size = 2,
          vjust = -0.5) +
facet_wrap(~drafted) +
theme_hc() +
ggtitle('40yrd Time Comparison of Draft Status by Position')
```

Creating a similar plot with `echarts4r` is a bit more involved. It is broken down into step-by-step code chunks and also requires an additional data object. The new data object `segments` compliments the existing `fortyYrd` object specific for line segments between the points.

In contrast to the base-R method demonstrated earlier a popular data manipulation package `dplyr` can employ the `group_by` function to perform a similar task. The `segments` object is declared by passing `fortyYrd` to `group_by` and now only the `Pos` variable. New calculations are then made for each position subset for the minimum, maximum, and the difference. The `summarise` get summary statistics from a grouped data set. This is then passed to `mutate` to create a new variable called `diff`. The end result is a four-column data frame, known as a "tibble" in the `dplyr` library, among others. This data ignores the aspect of draft status to calculate these statistics.

```
segments <- fortyYrd %>%
  group_by(Pos) %>%
  summarise(
    min = min(Forty.average),
    max = max(Forty.average)) %>%
  mutate(diff = max - min)
```

To improve the aesthetics of the visualization, let's sort by the segments by the minimum values before passing them to the `e_charts4r` functions. Both data frames are passed an `order` function to the left of a comma within square brackets. The `order` function will rearrange the rows by a numeric vector along with the parameter `decreasing=T`.

```
fortyYrd <- fortyYrd[order(fortyYrd$Forty.min, decreasing = T),]
segments <- segments[order(segments$min, decreasing = T),]
```

With both the `fortyYrd` and `segments` data, the visualization can be created. Using `echarts4r` has benefits in that it translates nicely to markdown dashboards explained elsewhere in the book. Static image libraries like `ggplot2` are explored in other chapters. Of course it is possible to reconstruct these images in other libraries but JavaScript dynamic plots will be illustrated for consistency. This code evolves slowly and is broken up into multiple chunks to create a Cleveland Dot Plot. To begin the `fortyYrd` data frame is forwarded using the pipe operator to `group_by` referring to the `drafted` column. Next, the `e_chart` is instantiated with *x*-axis declared as the `Pos` column. A scatter plot layer is then added with `e_scatter`. This layer requires the column `Forty.average` with an optional aesthetic parameter. Additional layers are added to provide mouse-over tooltips and a "save as" button. Ultimately this chart information is declared in the `p` object.

```
p <- fortyYrd %>%
  group_by(drafted) %>%
  e_charts(Pos) %>%
  e_scatter(Forty.average, symbol_size = 10) %>%
  e_tooltip(trigger = "item") %>%
  e_toolbox_feature(feature = "saveAsImage")
```

This visual is far from complete and another chunk must be added to the `p` object. One could put all these layers in series, but this can be complicated and it's a best practice until you are fluent to break up the effort into sections to ensure the code is error free. Once again, the chart is instantiated with `e_data` but now refers to the `segments` data with `Pos` to ensure the final components are positioned correctly. Next, the `e_bar` function adds a bar series to the plot. The complicated aspect is that the bars are made transparent with `rgba(0,0,0,0)`. This is a trick often employed in dot plots and waterfall charts. Transparent bars act as a background helping subsequent layers with labels to be placed correctly. In fact, this is the case for the visible segments layered next. You can observe these bars by changing the "rgba" section to simply "red." Doing so will ensure the bars show up so they can be seen although it ruins the visual effect!

```
p <- p %>%
  e_data(segments, Pos) %>%
  e_bar( # this bar goes from 0 to min average
    min,
    legend = FALSE,
    stack = "bars",
    itemStyle = list(
```

```
        barBorderColor = "rgba(0,0,0,0)",
        color = "rgba(0,0,0,0)"),
    emphasis = list(
    itemStyle = list(
        barBorderColor = "rgba(0,0,0,0)",
        color = "rgba(0,0,0,0)")))
```

Finally, another layer is added to create the visual line segments. The `p` object inherits another `e_bar` layer and refers to the latest data layer, `segment` with the `diff` column. The other parameters are straightforward and can be adjusted as needed. The `e_flip_coords` function merely switches *x/y* axes while `e_themes` can be adjusted to a more contrasting color combination as needed. Figure 4.10 is the final product of these lengthy codes. In the end, it is a dot plot with mouse-over tooltips demonstrating the average values for drafted and undrafted 40-yard times by position.

While further explanation may be warranted and additional visualizations can be constructed, the following code begins the Modify step within SEMMA. The `Round` variable ranges from 1 to 7 with NA. However, these are not integers. The values represented ordinal factors, because it is a class of athletes not a numeric value for the row. One modification may be to overwrite this variable with a character based factor to avoid confusion. Here, the `ordered` function is applied to the `Round` column. The existing levels are represented in the second parameter `c(1:7, "NA")`; the recoding occurs with the `labels` input and a string vector. The two latter inputs must correspond or be ordered so that 1 corresponds to "first," and so on. This modification needs to be applied to the

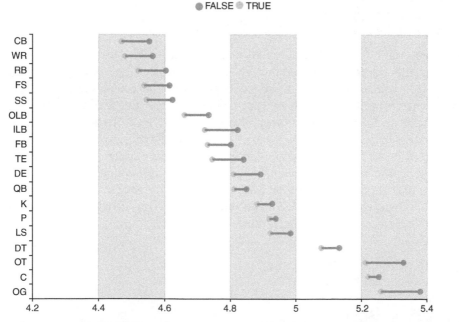

Figure 4.10 A barbell Dot Plot demonstrating the 40-yard sprint time differences between draft and undrafted athletes.

validation partition not just the training partition though is not shown below. It is not needed in the test partition because the 'Round' column has been removed making for a more realistic modeling experience. Team personnel would not have the most recent outcomes only historical data.

```
combineTraining$Round <- ordered(combineTraining$Round,
                           levels = c(1:7,'NA'),
                           labels = c('first', 'second',
                                      'third', 'fourth',
                                      'fifth','sixth',
                                      'seventh', 'NA'))
```

Additional modifications are needed depending on the machine learning algorithm chosen. The KNN algorithm measures distances; therefore, all inputs need to be numeric and scaled. There is no way to get a distance between "short" and "tall," for example. Instead, the height data needs to be numeric and scaled so it is relative to other numeric inputs. There are multiple methods to "clean" data. This may entail the creation of "dummy" variables where non-numeric data is represented as 1 or 0. An easy way to perform variable treatment is with the 'vtreat' package. This package accepts the data, builds a treatment plan, and then the plan is applied to existing or new data. To construct the variable treatment plan, the 'designTreatmentsZ' function accepts the data, or a partition, along with the names of the input variable columns. The package provides additional design treatment functionality for binary classification or numeric outcomes which require additional inputs. 'designTreatmentsZ' is demonstrated below for simplicity. Regardless of the design treatment used, dummy variables, imputation, and other common data-cleaning functions are understood within the plan that is then applied to data before modeling. First, 'informativeFeatures' is created using the 'names' function indexing only the specific input names. This creates a string vector of inputs. The data and input string vector are passed to 'designTreatmentsZ' to construct the data plan.

```
informativeFeatures <- names(combineTraining)[2:10]
variablePlan <- designTreatmentsZ(dframe = combineTraining,
                          varlist = informativeFeatures)
```

The 'prepare' function applies the learned treatment plan to the different data partitions 'combineTraining', 'combineValidation', and 'combineTest'. These cleaned partitions are held in new data frame objects 'treatedTraining', 'treatedValidation', and 'treatedTest'. The new objects now have 34 columns. Three major modifications have been applied to the data. First, an engineered variable 'Pos_catP' was made. This is a "prevalence fact" known as mean response encoding. Next, anytime a column contains NA the value is imputed with the mean average of the column. Additionally, when this occurs a binary column ending in '_isBad' is constructed. This retains the information that NA was corrected. Some algorithms can learn from this additional pattern information. Lastly, each level in the 'Pos' column has been turned into a series of dummy variables. For example, any wide receiver in the data set is now a 1 in the newly constructed 'Pos_lev_x_WR' column. For all others the value is 0. Creating dummy variables has occurred for all positions. These manipulations have meant the data has become wider but there is no new information or statistically risky adjustments that would undermine the model.

```
treatedTraining    <- prepare(variablePlan, combineTraining)
treatedValidation  <- prepare(variablePlan, combineValidation)
treatedTest        <- prepare(variablePlan, combineTest)
```

The last modification that is needed is to ensure the binary outcome variable is a factor type. R interprets Boolean values equivalent to 1 and 0. As a result, some modeling methods will not recognize the Boolean `drafted` column as distinct classes and instead infer the outcome is numeric or continuous. To ensure this is not the case, the `as.factor` function is applied to the original `drafted` column for each partition. The factored "TRUE" and "FALSE" are not distinct classes that will not be understood as 1 or 0. The modified vectors are appended to the corresponding treated partition as a new column on the left of the assignment operator.

```
treatedTraining$drafted    <- as.factor(combineTraining$drafted)
treatedValidation$drafted  <- as.factor(combineValidation$drafted)
treatedTest$drafted        <- as.factor(combineTest$drafted)
```

Moving to the modeling step of SEMMA, let's begin with the binary classification model construction. Remember the binary classification goal is to get ever player's probability of simply being drafted. As a scout, this could help you spend more time evaluating the most likely candidates, so this model could act as a triage for the scouting workload.

There are multiple applicable algorithms for binary classification. KNN is exemplified here but this code purposely employs the `train` function from `caret`. This makes changing the algorithm easy with a different `train` parameter along with different pre-processing methods.

The first input to `train` is a formula that sets up how the algorithm should be applied. The formula refers to column names of the data frame object within the `data` parameter. Here, the `drafted` column is the dependent variable. This variable depends on the *x*-variables as inputs. The formula could be explicitly defined as shown below:

```
drafted = Ht + Wt + Forty + … + Pos+lev_x_WR
```

However, since the data frame only contains the dependent variable and independent variables, as opposed to non-informative features like unique identifiers, the formula can be abbreviated with a period. Thus, the formula is `drafted ~ .`. The data frame, `treatedTraining`, is the next parameter followed by the method as a string, "KNN." The last two parameters are specific to the algorithm chosen. In this case, the data must be centered and scaled so an *x*-variable does not overwhelm the informative impact of the others. This can be the case when values differ greatly such as the `Shuttle` variable measured in seconds with single digits compared to the `Wt` which is in hundreds of pounds. A "scaled" data frame will take column means and subtract it from each individual column value. Then, the column values are divided by the standard deviation of the specific column. This measures the distance in standard deviations for each value. In doing so, all values are in the same scale, meaning 1 or 2 standard deviations from its column-wise counterparts. The last `tuneLength` parameter dictates the number of nearest neighbors to try when building the model. Although the number is even, the algorithm will try odd increments such as 3, 5, 7 until 20 odd nearest neighbors have been fit. Odd numbers are needed to avoid ties, where the nearest neighbors would dictate an exact 50% probability which is not practically helpful.

```
knnFit <- train(drafted ~ .,
                data = treatedTraining,
                method = "knn",
                preProcess = c("center","scale"),
                tuneLength = 20)
```

Moving to the "assess" phase of SEMMA, a simple way to evaluate the model fit is with `plot`. The resulting figure shown in Figure 4.11 shows the relationship between the nearest neighbors and overall accuracy. As the figure demonstrates, the number of neighbors increases the accuracy but there is a diminishing return. This plot and the subsequent assessments help to choose the correct number of neighbors. A `caret` model object will automatically select the *K*-value that maximizes accuracy even if the `tuneLength` was longer.

```
plot(knnFit)
```

Next, use the `predict` function with the KNN model and the two data partitions. This will select the most accurate *K*-value and use it on new records. KNN is a nonparametric model meaning instead of coefficients, the model must contain the original training data so that the new records can be scored according to the optimized *K*-value. The `predict` function is a generic function that can be applied to many modeling objects not just KNN. Thus, if the `method` parameter is changed in the `train` function, the

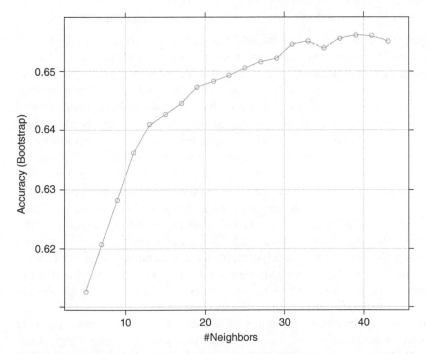

Figure 4.11 The neighbor to accuracy relationship demonstrating the diminishing relationship for the tuning parameter.

Table 4.6 The training set confusion matrix results.

		Reference/Actual outcomes	
		FALSE (not drafted)	TRUE (drafted)
Predicted classes	FALSE (not drafted)	490	263
	TRUE (drafted)	1534	3269

`predict` function is still applicable for scoring new records. As written this code will return the classification outcome assuming a 0.50 cutoff threshold. If probabilities for each class are needed, then an additional parameter within `predict` is needed. If this is the case, add a comma to denote the third input along with `type = "prob"` before closing out the `predict` function call.

```
trainingPreds   <- predict(knnFit, treatedTraining)
validationPreds <- predict(knnFit, treatedValidation)
```

Since the actual classifications were obtained, no additional steps are needed to calculate a confusion matrix. This matrix is a cross-tabulation of the model's classifications to the actual outcomes. One can call the `table` function or for more information utilize `caret`'s `confuctionMatrix` function. According to the documentation, the first parameter is the classified outcomes followed by the actual outcomes. Table 4.6 shows the basic tabular results.

```
confusionMatrix(trainingPreds, treatedTraining$drafted)
confusionMatrix(validationPreds, treatedValidation$drafted)
```

To understand the confusion matrix, the intersection of predicted and actual class levels on the diagonal represents the number of records that the model correctly classified. In the previous table, 490 athletes were predicted to be undrafted and were actually undrafted. Similarly, 3269 athletes were classified as drafted and were actually drafted. Thus, the overall model's accuracy is the sum of 490 and 3269 (correct classifications) divided by the entire matrix total, 490 + 263_1534 + 3269 which equals 5556, thus, 3759/5556 or 0.67. Keep in mind that a random sampling of records may have different results in the confusion matrix and that this assumes a 0.50 probability cutoff threshold.

If the cutoff threshold is changed, then the numbers populating the confusion matrix will change. For example, if the probability cutoff is 0.999 meaning only probabilities higher than this are classified as drafted, then no athletes would be in the predicted TRUE cell. The bar to being drafted would be exceedingly high. Conversely, if the threshold for a TRUE classification were 0.001, then all athletes would be considered TRUE. Besides pure accuracy with a 0.50 cutoff, one can iteratively adjust the cutoff value and record the changing relationship between the model's "sensitivity" and "specificity." Sensitivity measures how many relevant items are selected among all positive classifications. Conceptually, this measures the model's ability to correctly identify the positive class, TRUE. Specificity measures how many negative observations were selected among the actual negatives. A model can be highly specific, with a high cutoff threshold, so that when an athlete is considered a TRUE, then the actual is too. But if the threshold is too high, then the model will not be very sensitive; no athletes would be identified with 0.999, for example. Conversely, model can be sensitive by predicting all positive classes with a low cutoff threshold, but this means the model is not specific. It is merely selecting all athletes for the draft. Although these two cutoffs are extremes, the overall relationship between sensitivity and specificity can be visualized in a "receiver operator curve," ROC.

First, use the `roc` function on the predicted and actual values. In this code, the outcomes need to be declared first as logical values, not factor levels. Once Boolean the values are simply multiplied by 1 so that the TRUE is transformed to 1 and FALSE to 0. This allows the numeric ROC values to be calculated.

```
trainingROC <- roc(as.logical(treatedTraining$drafted)*1,
                   as.logical(trainingPreds)*1)
```

To visualize the relationship between sensitivity and specificity, call `plot` on the object. To interpret the ROC plot, understand that the darker line represents "model lift" over random. The diagonal line segments the visual into two equal components. This is like flipping a coin. The closer the line to the diagonal, the more likely the model is no better than flipping a coin. In fact a common classification key performance indicator, KPI, is call "area under the curve" representing the total area under the curve in this visual. Figure 4.12 shows the model's lift over random for the training data.

```
plot(trainingROC, main = 'Training ROC')
```

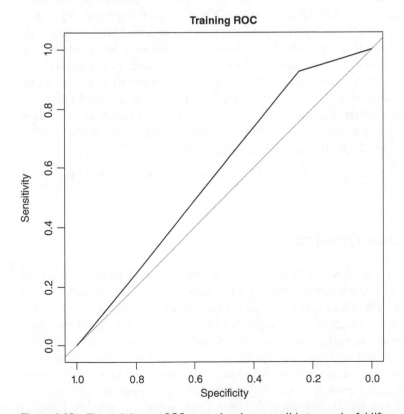

Figure 4.12 The training set ROC curve showing a small but meaningful lift over random guessing.

Table 4.7 Showing individual class probabilities which sum to 1 for each player row.

	FALSE	TRUE
Player1	0.609	0.390
Player2	0.390	0.609
Player3	0.585	0.414
Player4	0.195	0.804
Player5	0.585	0.414
Player6	0.073	0.926

These evaluation steps and visuals can be recreated with the other data partitions. In machine learning, the ability to "overfit" data is a serious concern. Models are optimized to fit the patterns in any data they are provided during the training step. The issue is that the model will not generalize to new unseen data which will undoubtedly be slightly different. Therefore, a model that overfits to the training data will be flawed or even useless in practice. Thus, rerun these assessments functions for the validation set looking for consistency for accuracy and model lift. Once the model demonstrates consistency, a new draft year's athletes can be confidently classified as draftable or not using the historical patterns learned by the model.

Other methods besides KNN could likely improve the model and accuracy outcomes though are more complex indicative of a traditional machine learning book. Regardless, when a stable model has been identified, predictions can be obtained for new data completely unseen in model training or validation. Keep in mind the new data needs to be in the same format as the original data and have the existing treatment plan applied so the model will accept it. For a realistic simulation of a draft where a section of potential athletes' actual outcomes are not known, the following code uses `predict` on the `treatedTest` partition. Further, the additional parameter to obtain probabilities has been added using the `type` parameter. Table 4.7 is the result of calling `head` on the `testPreds` to demonstrate the two column probability results.

```
testPreds <- predict(knnFit, treatedTest, type = 'prob')
head(testPreds)
```

Code—Multi-Class Classification

Another modeling approach would be to explicitly identify the round a player is expected to be chosen. This type of analysis may help identify when a player is over or under valued in the selection process. Recall that contracts are big for earlier round picks so having objective confirmation of a talent could be useful and more so a model classifying a low-round pick may temper an enthusiastic qualitative scouting report. A model like this will help inform decisions and improve efficient use of contract money and limited draft picks.

Rather than restarting the process, the following code applies the variable treatment plan to the original data partitions. This has the effect to drop the engineered `drafted` column so the new *y*-variable can be appended next. Thus, reapply the `prepare` function using the existing `variablePlan` to `combineTraining`, `combineValidation`, and `combineTest`.

```
treatedTraining    <- prepare(variablePlan, combineTraining)
treatedValidation <- prepare(variablePlan, combineValidation)
treatedTest        <- prepare(variablePlan, combineTest)
```

Next, the actual round classification variable from the partition is attached to the treated data forms. Recall the `Round` column was adjusted with `ordered` in the modification step. This must be applied across both training and validation observations. For more realistic modeling, the test set `Round` data has been removed from this data set. This mimics the knowledge a team may have for new athletes on any given year.

```
treatedTraining$Round    <- combineTraining$Round
treatedValidation$Round <- combineValidation$Round
```

There are two paths forward in this type of modeling exercise. On one hand, removing the NA values would improve the multiclass model results. However, it is not realistic because team personnel would not know if an athlete has been drafted or not when making these classifications. The model is needed for the entire draft cohort and the model determines the draft round, including if the athlete has a class level of "NA." Instead, a more realistic experience would be to treat the "NA" class as a factor level representing the information of an athlete that will not be drafted.

The following code treats the string `"NA"` as a factor with `as.factor`. This is represented on the right side of the assignment operator. On the left, the vector `Round` is indexed with `is.na`. When a value in the vector is NA, the function returns a TRUE, otherwise the value will remain. Thus, when TRUE, the not available NA value in the vector is changed to the *factor* type "NA." This is needed because R interprets NA as a particular type of class versus a piece of information relevant to the draft problem context.

```
treatedTraining$Round[is.na(treatedTraining$Round)]    <-
as.factor('NA')
treatedValidation$Round[is.na(treatedValidation$Round)] <-
as.factor('NA')
```

One of the benefits of KNN is that it can be used for multiclass problems. Once again, the nearest neighbors vote toward the probability. The difference is that relevant observations each contribute to multiple probabilities which sum to 1 rather than just the neighbors being of only one or another class levels. This code reapplies the `train` function from `caret`. In this case, the formula needs to be adjusted so that the `Round` variable depends on all other variables in the data object. The data parameter is still `treatedTraining` but recall the dependent variable is now `Round`. So, the code may look the same but the underlying object is different and the model will be too.

```
knnFit <- train(Round ~ .,
                data = treatedTraining,
                method = "knn",
                preProcess = c("center","scale"),
                tuneLength = 10)
```

Once again, the overall accuracy can be applied with `plot` on the model object. The issue with measuring overall accuracy is that this assumes there is an equal business impact to the "first" factor level compared to any other level including the "NA." This is clearly not the case because the cost of misclassifying a first-round draft pick as a second or third may mean the team is unable to draft a talented player. Perhaps worse is if a player that should be a seventh round or undrafted altogether gets misclassified as a highly talented first or second rounder. The contractual cost and wasted pick can have long-term repercussions for a team. Additionally, the overall accuracy may appear low, but in reality, among eight factor levels even a relatively low accuracy may be useful.

```
plot(knnFit)
```

To get more insight, first call `predict` using the model object and the data partitions. Once again the probabilities are not returned, only the 0.50 cutoff determined final class level is returned. If needed, the `type = "prob"` parameter can be employed in multi-class classifications.

```
trainingPreds   <- predict(knnFit, treatedTraining)
validationPreds <- predict(knnFit, treatedValidation)
```

As a result of the actual problem context, more examination must be done to assess the model starting with a more complex confusion matrix. The multiclass confusion matrix has eight rows and columns to intersect. The `confusionMatrix` is called below and also saved as an object `cm` for additional assessment. Table 4.8 shows the resulting multiclass matrix for the training set.

```
cm <- confusionMatrix(trainingPreds, treatedTraining$Round)
cm
```

As is often the case in typical business problems, the cost of a certain classification is more than other class levels. In a professional athlete draft, the first-round picks are very costly. Thus, the accuracy within this particular class requires additional scrutiny in comparison to other rounds.

Table 4.8 The training set confusion matrix with the diagonal, correctly classified observations highlighted.

		Reference/Actual outcomes							
		First	Second	Third	Fourth	Fifth	Sixth	Seventh	NA
	First	117	50	42	37	29	20	26	52
	Second	9	18	12	10	3	8	2	14
	Third	42	27	43	27	22	14	6	22
Predicted classes	Fourth	1	6	7	12	8	6	4	8
	Fifth	5	7	4	6	9	3	2	7
	Sixth	0	0	0	1	1	1	1	3
	Seventh	0	0	1	1	0	2	1	0
	NA	364	416	443	463	426	376	391	1918

The sensitivity of first-round draft classes is 0.218. This means about one in five actual first-round picks are being correctly identified. This may not be great because many top prospects are being overlooked by the model. However, this may also indicate that other athletes selected in the first round may not be truly elite. If the latter is the case, then a team would be well served to trade out of the first round because many of the first-round picks could easily be as talented as the other draft classes but at a fraction of the cost. Contextualizing this against the number of first-round "busts" where players are paid a huge first-round contract against their input to the team's outcome supports this hypothesis.

The code below selects just the `byClass` elements of the confusion matrix object showing these metrics. It is simple arithmetic to manually calculate the sensitivity. The numerator is 117, the true positive first-round class rate divided by the sum of the entire first-round class column (117 + 9 + 42 + 1 + 5 + 0 + 0 + 364).

```
cm$byClass
```

As before, if the model is acceptable within a sports management context, it can be applied to new data simulating a realistic draft day scenario where outcomes are not known. Otherwise, adjusting the number of neighbors or switching to a more complex model may be warranted. Assuming the exemplified model fits the business need, a prediction on new data is needed. The new data must be in the same initial format, be prepared with the existing variable treatment plan, and then the existing model object will accept it. The difference is that the `Round` column does not exist as it did in the training and validation partitions. Therefore, one cannot assess the model against this temporaneous data until time has passed and actuals are known.

```
testPreds <- predict(knnFit, treatedTest)
```

Code—Continuous Regression

KNN can also be applied with continuous supervised learning problems. Instead of the nearest neighbors each providing a vote resulting in a probability, the nearest K neighbors are averaged to make a prediction.

Once again, the code below reestablishes the data partitions without the *y* variable.

```
treatedTraining   <- prepare(variablePlan, combineTraining)
treatedValidation <- prepare(variablePlan, combineValidation)
treatedTest       <- prepare(variablePlan, combineTest)
```

Now, the `Pick` column is appended. Rather than a factor, the `Pick` column represents the draft order historically and is therefore numeric from 1 to 260. Although team needs and draft orders change from year to year, a model like this articulates the historical average draft pick number. If a team has a drastic need, they may ignore this model's output to fill a position gap, but this prediction may contextualize how much above or below they got particular player. Player personnel can judge for themselves if they believe they could wait despite a dire position need.

```
treatedTraining$Pick   <- combineTraining$Pick
treatedValidation$Pick <- combineValidation$Pick
```

Calling `summary` on the appended training set column notifies that the number of NAs is significant. Recall the NA represents when a player was not drafted. This model is predicting the draft order. As a result, imputing or replacing the NA by the mean or median will reinforce an incorrect data pattern. Thus, after calling `summary` the NA rows are removed. On the right of the assignment operator within each data frame object, a square bracket is used for indexing. Since the logical operator of `is.na` is to the left of the comma, the outcome will be applied to rows as opposed to columns. Of course `is.na` is not what is needed so the Boolean values are switched with `!`. When an NA value occurs in the `Pick` column, a TRUE is returned but switched to FALSE. The result is declared as the rows to drop in the entire data frame not just the single column that was evaluated.

```
summary(treatedTraining$Pick)
treatedTraining <- treatedTraining[!is.na(treatedTraining$Pick),]
treatedValidation <- treatedValidation[!is.na(treatedValidatio
n$Pick),]
```

In the previous KNN fits, a warning for zero variance variables was printed when calling `train`. This is a warning alerting the modeler that variables with 0 variances are contained in the training data which may impact the model. To remedy this before any of the `train` functions demonstrated previously, call the `nearZeroVar` from `caret` on the training data. Additionally, this step could be integrated into the modification step after extensive exploratory data analysis demonstrates the zero variances of certain columns. However, in practice this may be done later in the SEMMA workflow. The code below applies `nearZeroVar` to the `treatedTraining` object within the square brackets for indexing. To the right of the comma, the function is applied from the first column to all columns minus the last one. This is because the *y*-variable is the last column and should not be reviewed. The `ncol` function call makes the code robust so that the review extends to the number of columns minus one versus an explicit declaration such as `1:35`. The object `zeroVarIdx` is a numeric index of columns that have near or zero variance.

```
zeroVarIdx <- nearZeroVar(treatedTraining[,1:ncol(treatedTrain
ing)-1])
```

Next, use the index of offending columns with a minus sign to the right of the comma so that they are dropped. This code simply rewrites the existing object instead of creating a new duplicative object.

```
treatedTraining <- treatedTraining[,-zeroVarIdx]
```

Now that the NA values in the *y*-variable and zero variance columns have been removed, another `train` call will refit the KNN algorithm. The adjusted formula referring to `Pick` will automatically change the model's behavior to make predictions. To be clear while not a particularly useful algorithm, KNN can be applied broadly and the `caret` code does not need to be changed other than the formula.

```
knnFit <- train(Pick ~ .,
                data = treatedTraining,
                method = "knn",
                preProcess = c("center","scale"),
                tuneLength = 20)
```

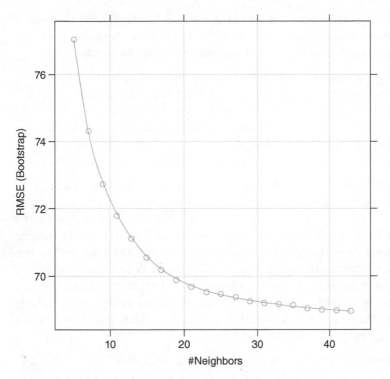

Figure 4.13   The error curve demonstrating that the RMSE error metric diminishes with more neighbors.

Previously the `plot` function showed a curve that wanted to be maximized. This is because it is a measure of accuracy which generally should be maximized. However, in regression problems, the root mean squared error, RMSE, is plotted. As an error metric, the goal is minimization not maximization. Usually as more neighbors are added, the curve slopes from upper left to lower right. Figure 4.13 shows a decreasing error rate with increasing neighbors but that has diminishing returns.

The RMSE metric is a useful KPI but is less commonsense compared to classification's accuracy. The RMSE first calculates the error. This is the difference from the actual and predicted values for all observations in the training set. The errors are then squared. Squaring the values ensures the predictions that are under the actual do not cancel out the error when the predicted values are above the actuals. Among all squared errors, the mean average is taken. Lastly, the square root of this value is calculated. Thus, the "root mean squared error" is merely worked in reverse of the acronym RMSE. The benefit of this metric is that the resulting error metric is in the units measured, meaning here that a RMSE of 66 is 66 actual draft picks. The model makes a single point prediction but may be off to the upside or downside by 66 picks. Of course, additional observations (rows) or new drill results (columns) along with different algorithms may improve results beyond this example.

After calling `predict` on both the `treatedTraining` and `treatedValida-tion` partitions, a simple data frame for each helps to stay organized for additional review. This code constructs `trainingResults` using `data.frame` where the first column is called `preds` referring to the predictions in `trainingPreds`. The second column, `picks`, is declared as the actual values of the training data. A similar data frame is constructed referring to the validation partition and corresponding actuals.

```
trainingPreds    <- predict(knnFit, treatedTraining)
validationPreds <- predict(knnFit, treatedValidation)
trainingResults <- data.frame(preds = trainingPreds,
                              picks = treatedTraining$Pick)
validationResults <- data.frame(preds = validationPreds,
                              picks = treatedValidation$Pick)
```

Many packages including `caret` have a `RMSE` function. Using the concise data frames, a comparison between partitions can be calculated with `RMSE`. The first input is the `preds` column and then the `picks`. When values like RMSE differ significantly between partitions, the model is likely overfitting or otherwise flawed. Here, the training RMSE is 66 and the validation RMSE is 69. These values are consistent if not good results. Thus, the model may be improved but is not structurally flawed. With a number this high, it is likely this model is regressing to the mean of the general population. In many cases, it may be improved by applying a recursive partition tree-based method or identifying additional column-wise data to supplement the rows. Still the KNN model can act as a baseline and is a useful algorithm for many objectives.

```
RMSE(trainingResults$preds, trainingResults$picks)
RMSE(validationResults$preds, validationResults$picks)
```

In the end, the validation set results are the most realistic assessment of the RMSE and model behavior since the model was constructed a priori. Assuming the test set has the same columns and is given the same treatment plan, the `knnFit` can be used with `predict` as below.

```
testPreds <- predict(knnFit, treatedTest)
```

Code–Unsupervised Learning (Clustering)

Finally, applying an unsupervised method, one can explore two clusters hopefully teasing out the draft status or by adding more clusters helping to tease out specific rounds. These methods rarely stand on their own but can supplement the supervised approaches. It is likely the case that some players identified as "drafted" also would-be part of a specific cluster or that some clusters are mostly made of first or second round draft picks confirmed with the multi-class model outcomes. The players exhibiting agreement despite approaches can help decision makers feel more comfortable in the analytical outcomes and recommendations. Thus, the *K*-means, *K*-medoid, and spherical *K*-means approaches can be used to affirm player level outputs of the pervious methods.

Transitioning to an unsupervised set of methods, let's reload the original data frame. The SEMMA approach could be recreated as before but this chapter's section will focus mostly on the clustering method and assessment to hopefully aid decision makers.

```
NFLcombineFile <- 'https://raw.githubusercontent.com/kwartler/
Practical_Sports_Analytics/main/C4_Data/combine_data_2000_
2020.csv'
NFLcombineFile <- getURL(NFLcombineFile)
NFLcombine <- read.csv(text = NFLcombineFile)
```

Since there is no manner to determine a distance with factors or strings, the first modification step would be to remove non-numeric columns. The `c` function creates a vector of column names to be removed. The `keeps` vector is then used while indexing `NFLcombine`. The `%in%` operator will create a Boolean response when the `keeps` column names are found `%in%` complete `names` vector of column strings. This logical response is to the right of the comma so that it applies to columns. The result is a smaller data frame of just numeric vectors called `numericData`.

```
keeps <- c('Ht', 'Wt','Forty','Vertical','BenchReps','BroadJump',
           'Cone','Shuttle','Round','Pick')

numericData <- NFLcombine[,names(NFLcombine) %in% keeps]
```

Another modification step that is needed is to deal with NAs. One could perform imputation by filling in the mean values for NA. However, this may skew a clustering technique measuring the mean. Instead, this code uses `complete.cases` indexing to the left of the comma. This will create a Boolean vector evaluating each row. If one or more NAs are identified, `complete.cases` will return a FALSE. The resulting `complete.cases` object will not contain any NA values and therefore will be accepted in the clustering functions.

```
completeCases <- numericData[complete.cases(numericData),]
```

As a distance-based approach, the data needs to be scaled. Applying the `scale` function will subtract the mean and divide by the standard deviation for each vector. This standardizes the data frame to the same unit of measure, the distance from mean measured in standard deviations for the column.

```
scaledCases <- scale(completeCases)
```

There are a total of seven rounds within the `Round` column. The code below will fit seven clusters as the second parameter of the `kmeans` function. The resulting cluster model object is a complex list object for assessment.

```
kmeanFit <- kmeans(scaledCases, 7)
```

To begin, let's examine the number of players within each cluster. This can be obtained in two manners, an object element called `size` is a vector of the cluster sizes. Similarly, a tabulation of the raw cluster assignments will yield the same results. In either case, the result is a frequency count of the observations' cluster assignment.

```
kmeanFit$size
table(kmeanFit$cluster)
```

Examining the averages within each cluster can be useful to contextualize it. To obtain the centers call the `centers` object element. It will be difficult to interpret since the data was scaled.

```
kmeanFit$centers
```

Since the values are scaled, the column standard deviations need to be multiplied and the column averages added to each value. This will back-transform the standardization. Luckily, this data is retained as attributes of the scaled data. The code below utilizes a custom function that is then applied. `backTransform` accepts a column to be readjusted. This is first multiplied by the attribute using `attr` referring to the scaled matrix. The second parameter is the name of the attribute representing the standard deviation, `scaled:scale`. This value is added to another original column attribute value. The `attr` function along with the scaled matrix and the `scaled:center` string refers to the columns average.

```
backTransform <- function(scaledCol){
 response <- scaledCol *
  attr(scaledCases, 'scaled:scale') +
  attr(scaledCases,
      'scaled:center')
  return(response)
}
```

Once instantiated, the `apply` function with margin `1` refers to rows of the scaled `centers` of the cluster object. For each row, the `backTransform` function is applied. In order to get the centers into the same shape as the original centers data, the entire code is nested in `t` to transpose it. The result is ` backCenters` a standalone object with values back-transformed for contextualization by the data professional. Upon close review, two clusters appear to be taller and heavier than others with `Ht` and `Wt` greater than 76 and 310, respectively. Some additional clusters have both shorter athletes but faster 40 times. The specific cluster numeric assignment, 1–7, may as the model converges but the underlying average centers will not adjust considerably.

```
backMeanCenters <- t(apply(kmeanFit$centers, 1, backTransform))
```

There are additional KPI related to cluster methods and even plots like a silhouette plot which helps optimize a cluster algorithm's number of clusters. Primarily, the within-ness and between-ness of the clusters described below are the basic starting points. Each can be called with the code below.

```
kmeanFit$withinss
kmeanFit$betweenss
```

- Within-ness is the sum of squared distance each data point has to the cluster centroid. As a distance measure for the tightness of the cluster, a lower value is better. When the value is high, there may be outliers affecting the center placement or that the number of clusters should be increased.
- Between-ness is the sum of squared distance between.

Often a single clustering method may not be the best. The code below will apply the `pam` function which will "partition around medoids" instead of mean averages.

```
kmedFit <- pam(scaledCases, 7)
```

Once again, the `backTransform` function can help rescale the centers. In this case, the centers are actually medoids representing the median values. Additionally, with this code the specific median athlete representing the prototypical cluster is returned as a row attribute. The second code line obtains these seven prototypical athletes from the original data set. For example, Leterrius Walton is one such player from among the large player clusters with a height of 77 inches and weight of 319 pounds. Since the data was reduced previously, the `kmedFit$id.med` element has the wrong row index. If the training data was not reduced, this element can be useful for identifying the prototypical observations.

```
backMedianCenters <- t(apply(kmedFit$medoids, 1, backTransform))
NFLcombine[rownames(backMedianCenters),]
```

The cluster size, distance to other clusters, and diameter in the hyperspace can be easily obtained with the `clusinfo` element. In this table, each cluster will have a simple count of observations. Additionally, the `max_diss` column is a measure of the entire internal cluster range, like measuring from one side of a state to another at the widest section. Next, the `av_diss` represents the average distance between points within the cluster. An analog is measuring the average distance between cities within a state. The `diameter` is a measure of the cluster's boarder. Lastly, the `separation` column is the distance among the clusters similar to the distance between states. Table 4.9 shows a rounded version of the cluster information element.

```
kmedFit$clusinfo
```

Lastly, applying the `skmeans` function will create spherical K-means based on cosine similarity not Euclidean distances. The second parameter represents the number of clusters. The `m` input is the hardness of the cluster boarder. This will help ensure some separation versus a "fuzzy" border where records are not clearly assigned a cluster.

```
skMeansFit <- skmeans(scaledCases,
                      7,
                      m = 1)
```

The centers are called `prototypes` in the modeling object. They need to be transformed as before using `backTransform`. Unlike the median analysis, these values

Table 4.9 The median cluster summary statistics.

Size	Max distance	Average distance	Diameter	Separation
189	3.66	1.90	5.93	0.64
342	3.90	1.73	5.87	0.60
285	3.20	1.77	5.29	0.64
268	2.97	1.73	5.24	0.62
350	4.12	1.94	6.52	0.78
228	3.60	1.82	6.14	0.60
160	3.05	1.73	5.31	0.64

will not be a specific player but the cosine similarity center of a cluster among the player statistics. Although the spherical K-means approach is well suited for sparse data like document text clustering, reviewing even the `Ht` and `Wt` prototypes demonstrates less extreme values.

```
backSKmeansCenters <- t(apply(skMeansFit$prototypes, 1,
backTransform))
```

One additional way to contextualize the clusters if by reviewing the proportion of a cluster's assignment to the actual draft round. Although the cluster assignments are 1–7, the numbers will not necessarily correspond to the `Round` column. This is because each clustering method arbitrarily assigns an integer as an identifier not corresponding to the information of `Round`. To begin, recreate the subset data but negate the Boolean result of `%in%`. Then apply the same `complete.cases` function call with `numericData` to ensure the rows match. This will retain the non-numeric rows which were complete numerically and as a result used in model training.

```
playerInfo <- NFLcombine[, !names(NFLcombine) %in% keeps]
playerInfo <- playerInfo[complete.cases(numericData),]
```

Once the non-numeric data has been aligned to the training data, each model's cluster assignment is appended to the data set. The *K*-means object refers to the `cluster` element. The *K*-medoid algorithm's cluster assignments are contained in `clustering`. The spherical *K*-means object refers to `cluster` for assignments. The code below refers to each and assigns a descriptive new column to the non-numeric data.

```
playerInfo$kMeansAssignment <- kmeanFit$cluster
playerInfo$kmedAssignment   <- kmedFit$clustering
playerInfo$skMeanAssignment <- skMeansFit$cluster
```

Lastly, the actual `Round` information is appended referring to the original `completeCases` object.

```
playerInfo$actualRound <- completeCases$Round
```

Once the data is organized, tabulating the proportion of a cluster assignment to a round is straightforward. First, call `table` referring to a specific cluster identifier and then the `actualRound` column. For example, this code first creates a table using `kMeansAssignment` and then the other methods' assignments.

```
KMeanTable  <- table(playerInfo$kMeansAssignment,
                     playerInfo$actualRound)
KMedTable   <- table(playerInfo$kmedAssignment,
                     playerInfo$actualRound)
skMeanTable <- table(playerInfo$skMeanAssignment,
                     playerInfo$actualRound)
```

These tables can be reviewed as row-wise proportions with `prop.table`. Since the `actualRound` variable is the second input to `table`, the margin parameter is 1 so that proportionality is calculated by row. To avoid excessive floating-point numbers,

Table 4.10 The Mediod cluster assignments as a proportion of the actual round selection.

		Actual draft round						
		1	2	3	4	5	6	7
	Cluster1	0.00	0.00	0.00	0.10	0.30	0.32	0.28
	Cluster2	0.14	0.23	0.31	0.27	0.05	0.00	0.00
	Cluster3	0.00	0.00	0.00	0.02	0.33	0.35	0.29
Cluster assignment	Cluster4	0.01	0.10	0.23	0.37	0.27	0.02	0.00
	Cluster5	0.22	0.25	0.25	0.22	0.06	0.00	0.00
	Cluster6	0.41	0.33	0.19	0.06	0.00	0.00	0.00
	Cluster7	0.00	0.00	0.00	0.00	0.02	0.33	0.65

the tabulation is nested in `round` with a parameter of `2` so decimals are limited to two places.

```
round(prop.table(KMeanTable,1),2)
round(prop.table(KMedTable,1),2)
round(prop.table(skMeanTable,1),2)
```

As previously discussed, the cost of first round is considerably higher than other rounds. As a result, the clustering method that best identifies the top first and second rounds is likely the most impactful to the business decision. Table 4.10 is the result of the K-medoid tabulation and proportional calculation. In this example, cluster assignment 6 has the highest concentration of actual round selection one. When rerunning the code, the assignment identifiers and proportions may differ slightly. Among the three methods, this method may be best suited for identifying top prospects. A comparison of proportional tables is needed by adjusting the previous code.

Since the Mediod method appears to identify the first-round draft picks best when the round is included, the model should be selected and refit without the round or pick information. This allows it to be employed ahead of the actual round. While the example demonstrates target leakage as written the exercise is meant to identify the best method for the business context, then a refit with correct variables can be performed. As written, this is easy by adjusting the `keeps` object. Once refit, new player evaluations need to be scaled according to the training data attributes. Small adjustments to the `backTransform` function will enable this scaling according to the training data. Once these steps are performed, the refit *K*-medoid object can be applied to identify top prospects.

Extending the Approaches Employed

There are multiple ways to extend the lessons of this chapter. For example, the data itself can be enriched. Not only are the player evaluations here reviewed by scouts but also regular season statistics, age at the time of the draft, and other factors like the college attended may play a role in professional success. As a result, it is worthwhile to enrich the data with other pertinent information. To do so, other open-source player data sets would be needed and various joins performed.

Another way to extend this chapter is by applying other classification methods. Supervised algorithms like decision trees, random forests, or Extreme Gradient Boosted Trees, known as XGB, can greatly enhance the accuracy and effectiveness of the model beyond the demonstration here. To employ other models, further exploration among `caret` package methods is required.

Similarly, there are other unsupervised algorithms that could yield different and possibly improved results. Some of the more popular methods include K-means and K-mediod clustering. The "K" parameters in each represent a tuning parameter the analyst should employ. This chapter focused on spherical K-means to demonstrate a less documented yet valuable tool in the data science tool kit.

Exercises

1) Describe the difference between supervised learning, in this case classification, and an unsupervised clustering technique such as spherical K-means.

2) List five potential data enrichment possibilities to improve the modeling outcome.

3) Create a scatter plot with $x = ...$ and $y =$ color coded by player position. Describe any pattern and what this may mean in terms of identifying signal in the data.

4) Change the `tuneLength` parameter to 10 for the binary classification KNN model. Plot the resulting KNN fit and describe the outcome.

5) Using the `tuneLength= 10` *binary* KNN model created in #4, predict the 2020 draft probabilities for each player.
   a) Sort the player draft probabilities in descending order. What are the top six most likely to be drafted?
   b) Calculate the accuracy, sensitivity, and specificity along with the confusion matrix for the validation set.

6) Change the `tunelength` for the *multi-class* KNN model to 10. Plot the modeling object and describe the visualization.

7) Using the multi-class `tunelength` KNN created in #6, print the confusion matrix.

8) Using the multi-class `tunelength` KNN created in #6, make predictions on the *validation partition*. Organize the data into a simple data frame with columns for player names, years, actual draft round, and predicted draft round.

a) Identify a single player that is overrated, one that went in a high round but the model classified as lower.

b) Identify a single player that is underrated, one that the model classified as an early draft pick but was not selected until later in reality.

9) Create a KNN regression model with `tuneLength` 10, assess the model's RMSE and score all data partitions.

10) Create a spherical *K*-means cluster using all the data and identify the prototypical athlete for the cluster with the largest number of athletes.

5

Logistic Regression

Explaining Basketball Wins and Losses with Coefficients

Objectives

- Follow the SEMMA approach to modeling
- Construct various visuals within the data exploration phase of the modeling exercise
- Build a logistic regression to model winning team characteristics
- Calculate multiple model key performance indicators and compare them across training and validation partitions
- Construct a waterfall using the model coefficients to understand the proportion of the model's output is explained by each feature
- Organize the modeling coefficients and winning team data to construct a scatter plot
- Interpret the scatter plot quadrants as a means to understand team behavior and what aspects of women's collegiate basketball should be focused or deprioritized by players and coaches
- Identify top-performing teams according to statistic(s) that may be overlooked by other teams

R Libraries

```
RCurl
ggplot2
ggthemes
echarts4r
MLmetrics
vcd
yardstick
waterfalls
```

Sports Analytics in Practice with R, First Edition. Ted Kwartler.
© 2022 John Wiley & Sons Ltd. Published 2022 by John Wiley & Sons Ltd.

R Functions

```
library
<-
getURL
read.csv
set.seed
sample
summary
ggplot
aes
geom_density
theme_hc
ggtitle
%>%
e_charts
e_density
e_toolbox_feature
e_theme
e_tooltip
ifelse
table
glm
predict
data.frame
geom_vline
LogLoss
Accuracy
table
sum
diag
autoplot
Kappa
print
coefficients
proportions
round
waterfall
subset
head
apply
rownames
match
names
```

```
for
length
paste
mean
max
min
geom_point
geom_text
geom_hline
annotate
```

Sports Context

This chapter seeks to quantitively explain the features of women's winning basketball teams. Keep in mind, there are different modeling purposes within machine learning. On one hand, a focus for predictive accuracy may lead to "black-box" or hard to interpret algorithms. This type of modeling exercise is useful when the cost or benefit is high and there is no need to understand the reason behind a model's output. In that case, focus on the accuracy or other model metric alone. On the other hand, there are times that models can be useful as diagnostic tools to explain a scenario. For some model types and outputs, there is an explanatory aspect which can help decision makers. This chapter focuses on explaining a basketball phenomenon. More specifically, this chapter will model the likelihood a team has a winning percentage above the third quartile among collegiate Women's Division I basketball teams. It would be of little use to create a highly accurate non-interpretable model to predict the overall outcome because this prediction represents an entire season. Knowing before game one of the seasons, the likelihood of a team's seasonal success without knowing why does not help a coach or player strategy.

Instead, the goal of this chapter is to use a logistic regression and examine the coefficients of the model in detail in order to identify basketball actions to prioritize, maintain, and even avoid. In the code example, a basketball action is measured in an offensive statistic while the exercises section asks the reader to recreate the analysis for defensive statistics. The hope is that a coach or player would know ahead of the season what to focus on during practices to improve the probability that over the course of a season they may have a top quartile winning percentage.

There is a data caveat for this chapter. The data was obtained using a web-scraping script posted to the book repository at the URL below. At the time of data collection, the scraped website had data integrity issues and offset HTML tables. Care was taken to correct the inconsistencies though other issues may remain. Further, perhaps because the level of detail is not as vigorous for female sports, many of the table results had incomplete observations. A straightforward imputation method was employed to complete some records, again available within the script website below. In the end, the data is sufficient for insights and learning but could be expanded and improved upon further.

> At the time of data collection, the script at this URL was used to construct the data. https://github.com/kwartler/Practical_Sports_Analytics/blob/main/C5_Data/final_ESPN.R

The data dictionary is as follows. All data are summarized at the seasonal team level as opposed to individual game or player:

- `NAME`—A factor level representing a Women's Division I basketball team university.
- `yr`—The integer year the season ended for the observation.
- `win`—An integer for the total number of wins a team had in a season.
- `loss`—An integer for the total number of losses a team had in a season.
- `PPG`—The "points per game" which is a numeric mean average for total points scored in a season divided by the total games in a season. This number is multiplied by 100.
- `FG_PCT`—The "field goal percentage" which is a numeric measure of how well a team shoots during the season. It is the total number of made shots divided by the total attempted. This value is multiplied by 100. The field goal percentage *does* include the three-point shots.
- `Three_Pt_FG_PCT`—A *subset* of the `FG_PCT` percentage accounting for shots taken in three-point range that are made divided by attempted three-points shots in a season. This value is multiplied by 100.
- `FT_PCT`—After a shooting foul, a player is able to take a free throw. The `FT_PCT` statistics is the number of free throws made divided by the total number of attempts in a season. This value is multiplied by 100. This statistic is *not included as part* of the field goal percentage.
- `Rebounds_PG`—The numeric rebounds per game where the total seasonal rebounds for a season are divided by the total number of games. For the coded example, the rebounds represent *only offensive rebounds*. In the exercises using the defensive data, the rebounds represent defensive rebounds only.
- `Assists_PG`—The numeric assists per game where the total seasonal number of assists are divided by the total number of games.

Technical Context

The major technical component of this chapter is the logistic regression built with `glm`. Recall the goal is to identify elite teams by regular season winning, as opposed to post season play, using the explanatory power of a model. The modeling problem is set up with a binary outcome where teams in the top quartile of winning percentage are assigned a TRUE, otherwise FALSE. This setup makes the exercise useful for the logistic regression. One could explore a similar exploratory case by restructuring the problem to be continuous. For example, a simple ordinary least squares regression could be fit on the `win` column which is continuous in nature.

However, the logistic regression model type is appropriate because the dependent or outcome variable is binary, meaning it has two states of nature such as TRUE or FALSE. A logistic regression has some similarities to a linear regression. Both are fit using a dependent variable usually called a target or "y" variable. Having a target makes the modeling effort a "supervised" exercise. Other chapters in the book demonstrate both supervised machine learning and unsupervised clustering techniques. This chapter only focuses on a single supervised approach to gain insight. Associated with each *y*-variable outcome is a series of *x*-variables. These inputs or informative features are expected to have some relationship to the *y*-variable. The logistic regression will seek to identify a linear relationship or pattern for each input that relates to the *y*-outcome variable. Unlike linear regression, in order for a logistic regression to be fit, the outcome is transformed. The outcome is changed to the "log-odds" of an observation being TRUE, not the numeric representation of TRUE, 1. Thus, the model is setup to actually find the linear combination of inputs to predict the *log-odds* of an event occurring not the event itself. Log-odds are not that intuitive, so the output is usually changed to a probability measure between 0 and 1. Although this chapter does use the probability a bit, the coefficients themselves and the accompanying data are examined closely rather than an individual team's output. In R, one can obtain either the log-odds of an event or the probability with the `predict` function. This is done by adjusting a parameter in the function call. To manually convert log-odds to probabilities, a simple equation is employed using "Euler's number" or "e." To observe the difference, consider the following code. The `probs` object contains the probabilities from a `fit` logistic regression. In contrast, the `rawP` object is the log-odds of an event as predicted with the `link` parameter.

```
probs  <- predict(fit, trainingData[1:10,5:11], type = 'response')
rawLog <- predict(fit, trainingData[1:10,5:11], type = 'link')
```

The `e` variable is declared as a floating-point number, specifically "Euler's number." However, this is an irrational number so the number conversion will not be exact since the `e` variable is not out to 64 decimal places. To convert the log-odds to probabilities, take `e` and raise it by the log-odds output from the logistic regression. This is divided by 1 plus the `e` raised to the log-odds. The preceding code and following conversion can be attempted within this chapter's case for exploration and improving technical acumen.

```
e <- 2.71828
e^rawP /(1+ e^rawP )
```

Code- Explaining Complexity with a Model's Parameters

To begin, let's download the data. As shown throughout the book, the `getURL` function is applied to the raw git repository URL string. Then `read.csv` is applied to the downloaded information. The result is a data frame of 550 records called `bbData`. Each row represents a collegiate Women's Division I basketball team for a season. Columns of the data set represent the college name, season ending year, and, in this example, offensive statistics. Within the repository there is another women's basketball data set specific for defensive statistics. Table 5.1 is a portion of the data to be explored and modeled.

```
bbData <- 'https://raw.githubusercontent.com/kwartler/Practical_
Sports_Analytics/main/C5_Data/imputed_OffensiveStats.csv'
```

Table 5.1 A portion of the women's basketball data.

Name	Yr	Win	Loss	PPG	FG_PCT	Three_Pt_ FG_PCT	FT_PCT	Rebounds_PG	Assists_PG
Notre Dame	2020	29	5	77.3	45.4	38.7	74.9	41.7	18.2
Missouri St.	2020	22	10	76.8	43.5	36.9	75.8	44.1	15.0
North Carolina	2020	19	12	76.5	43.2	35.8	75.3	46.8	15.4

```
offensiveStats <- getURL(bbData)
offensiveStats <- read.csv(text = offensiveStats)
```

In machine learning applications, there is a need to sample to avoid overfitting. Algorithms will over-learn patterns in the data. The result is a model that performs well on data used during training but generalizes poorly when presented to new data. The learned patterns are said to be "over fit." To avoid this problem, a simple workflow called SEMMA demonstrated here and in this chapter regarding player evaluations dictates that the data must be sampled. In fact, SEMMA stands for Sample, Explore, Modify, Model, and Assess. First, `set.seed` is applied only for educational purposed. Setting a non-random seed means when random number generation is enacted, the result will be consistent. Here, this ensures the subsequent visuals and model are consistent to the example chapter. Next, `sample` is applied to obtain a vector of randomly generated numbers. The vector to be samples ranges from one to the `nrow` or number of rows within the data set. While one could explicitly declare `1:550` it is a best practice to make the code dynamic as data set size may change. The second input dictates the number of selections to make. The `size` parameter is merely the number of rows, 550, times 0.8 or 440. The `idx` object is a vector of 440 integers between 1 and 550 that are randomly selected. This is used within square brackets to the left of the comma to create `trainingData` and with a `-idx` to declare the remaining 110 rows as the `validationData`. Thus, the model will be fit using training data, as compared to the known results of the validation set. The goal is consistent performance among the partitions which should indicate the model is *not* overfit.

```
set.seed(1234)
idx <- sample(1:nrow(offensiveStats), nrow(offensiveStats) *.8)
trainingData <- offensiveStats[idx,]
validationData <- offensiveStats[-idx,]
```

Now that the data is sampled, the "Explore" step is next. Exploratory Data Analysis or EDA is a major yet often overlooked aspect of modeling. This helps the practitioner first establish the data is as expected such as queried from a data base correctly and secondarily helps identify nuances or interesting insights. First, call `summary` on the training data frame. This will print vector level information. Most notably one would notice there are six statistical numeric vectors. The `summary` call provides minimum, quartile, median, mean, and maximum values. Had the data set contained missing NA values, the count is also returned. However, this data has already been reduced to exclude incomplete records.

```
summary(trainingData)
```

Next, it is a good idea to visualize the distribution of variables. The code below demonstrates the construction of a kernel density plot using `ggplot`. A kernel density plot is similar to a histogram, but it smooths the plot values. The tallest point of the kernel density plot displays the most numerous or concentrated values. First, pass in the data frame to `ggplot` along with the aesthetics parameter declaring the *x*-axis as `PPG` vector. Next, declare the plot type with `geom_density`, add a theme from High Charts with `theme_hc`. Lastly, add a simple title with a string passed to the last layer using `ggtitle`. Figure 5.1 is the result of the code. In practice one would explore more than a single points per game statistic to ensure consistency with expectations or identify outliers to be removed.

```
ggplot(trainingData, aes(x = PPG)) +
  geom_density() +
  theme_hc() +
  ggtitle('Points Per Game')
```

The same density plot can be constructed with `echarts4r`. Here the `training-Data` is piped to `e_charts` to instantiate a blank type. This is forwarded to `e_density` to setup the visual. The statistic column has been changed to `Assists_PG` along with a title parameter and some aesthetic inputs. The last three layers add user functionality to download a static image, change the overall colors to gray theme, and add a mouseover tooltip.

```
trainingData %>%
  e_charts() %>%
  e_density(Assists_PG,
            name = "Assists_PG Density",
            areaStyle = list(opacity = .4),
            smooth = TRUE) %>%
  e_toolbox_feature(feature = "saveAsImage") %>%
  e_theme('gray') %>%
e_tooltip()
```

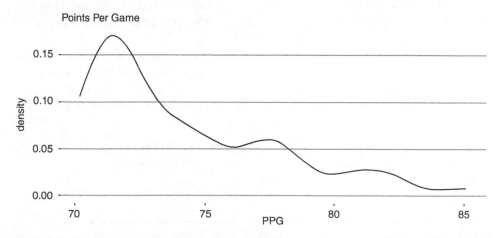

Figure 5.1 The PPG kernel density plot showing the most numerous value is ~72 (the highest point).

A calculation is needed to identify top performing regular season teams. The `winning Pct` object calculates the winning percentage for each team in the data set. This is the number of wins divided by the sum of both wins and losses. This simple calculation is nested inside of `summary`. Since the data has been prepared to remove the records with missing data, there is a propensity to retain teams from successful programs. Effectively there is a selection bias in that major, successful teams are more likely to have complete records and were therefore retained. To account for this, a successful team has been defined as any value higher than the third quartile. In the end, these teams represent the best of the best, accounting for likely selection bias in the underlying data. The `third-Quartile` object is a single dynamically declared value but with more complete data from other sports or programs could be adjusted lower while still encompassing high performing teams.

```
winningPct <- summary(trainingData$win/(trainingData$win+train
ingData$loss))
thirdQuartile <- winningPct[5]
```

Moving to the next "Modify" step in the process, the code section engineers a dependent variable. Using a control operator `ifelse`, a Boolean response is created as a new variable declared on the left of the assignment operator called `winningSeason`. The logical check is whether or not a team's individual winning percentage, calculated as `win` divided by sum of `win` and `loss`, is greater than the `thirdQuartile` value previously calculated. As sports and data sets change, this value could be adjusted. For example, in collegiate men's basketball, a simple 0.50 winning percentage may yield acceptable insights. The logical construction is applied to both the `trainingData` and `validationData`.

```
trainingData$winningSeason <- ifelse((trainingData$win /
(trainingData$win + trainingData$loss)>thirdQuartile), T, F)
```

```
validationData$winningSeason <- ifelse((validationData$win /
(validationData$win + validationData$loss)>thirdQuartile), T, F)
```

With the *y*-variable calculated, a simple `table` call will illustrate the distribution of the elite versus non-elite regular season winning teams. Table 5.2 is the tally of the TRUE and FALSE results.table(trainingData$winningSeason)

The next step is to actually train a model on the data. To train a logistic regression, the `glm` function is applied. The `glm` model fits generalized linear models. It first accepts a formula-based representation. In this case, the `winninSeason` variable is within `as.factor` and declared as the dependent variable. Often using `as.factor` is not needed

Table 5.2 The approximate three-to-one ratio among team winning percentages.

FALSE	TRUE
Teams with winning percentage < third quartile	Teams with winning percentage > third quartile
333	107

but is considered a sound practice particularly with algorithms that can be applied to continuous and classification such as random forest. Next, the tilda, `~`, begins the right side of the equation where each independent variable is listed. As a shortcut a simple period instructs the `glm` to accept all other columns as informative features. This is only appropriate if it is true, so be careful the period does not end up including non-*x*-variables like `yr`, `NAME`, or unique identifiers. In the code below, this is accomplished by limiting the data parameter to only columns `5:11` which represent the statistics of interest. Lastly, the `glm` function needs a `family` parameter. There are multiple possible inputs dependent on the distribution of the *y*-variable and the modeling task. Here, `binomial` represents the logit link for a logistic regression.

```
fit <- glm(as.factor(winningSeason)~.,
           trainingData[,5:11],
           family = 'binomial')
```

The last and most informative aspect of the SEMMA workflow is "Assess." In order to assess the model's behavior, predictions must be made. Rather than obtain the log-odds of an outcome, the probability is obtained with the code below. The `preds` vector of probabilities is obtained using `predict`. The first parameter is the model object and the second is the data to be scored. This is an in-sample prediction since it is the values for training data. The last parameter set to `response` ensures the results are returned as probabilities between 0 and 1.

```
preds <- predict(fit, trainingData[,5:11], type = 'response')
```

Next, let's create the actual classification and organize the in-sample model results into a simple data fame. First, declare a cutoff value. Depending on the use case, 0.5 may not be appropriate. For example, in direct mail identifying the most likely respondents is important so a higher cutoff threshold would be appropriate. In this case, the dependent variable represents elite teams at the third quartile of winning percentage. Therefore, the standard 0.5 is acceptable. The `plotDF` is constructed with `data.frame` and three declared vectors. The first `preds` is simply the raw probability scores. Next, the actual outcomes from the training data are added. Finally, the `class` or classified outcome is instantiated using another `ifelse` to logically check whether the prediction probabilities are above the previously declared cutoff.

```
cutoff <- 0.5
plotDF <- data.frame(preds = preds,
                     actual = trainingData$winningSeason,
                     class = ifelse(preds>=cutoff,T,F))
```

One way to observe model behavior is visualizing the distribution of probabilities for the success and failure classes. Ideally there is a separation of the two cohorts at the cutoff threshold. This would mean the model has successfully identified patterns in the data denoting success and failures. To do so, pass the `plotDF` data to `ggplot`. The aesthetics declare the `preds` column as the *x*-axis. No *y*-axis is needed since the code is constructing a kernel density plot. The color parameter and line types refer to the `actual` column so that the line's color and solid versus dashed look are inherited from the true values of the data. The next layer instantiates the kernel density plot with `geom_density`. The parameter inside this layer merely declares a consistent line thickness for easier interpretation but is optional. An additional layer is added using `geom_vline` to append a vertical line starting at the 0.50 `cutoff` value declared earlier along with a bold color. The last two layers simply change the aesthetics and add a title which are likely straightforward at this point in this chapter. The resulting plot, captured in Figure 5.2, shows a reasonable separation of the two actual classes.

```
ggplot(plotDF, aes(x=preds, color=actual, linetype=actual)) +
  geom_density(size = 1.25) +
  geom_vline(aes(xintercept = cutoff), color = 'black') +
  theme_hc() +
  ggtitle('Probability Density w/Cutoff Eliminating Majority
  of Losing Teams')
```

Notice in Figure 5.2, the majority of FALSE, non-elite teams, are on the left of the cutoff. Although the probability likelihoods for the elite teams are relatively flat, the majority are slightly more on the right-hand side of the vertical line. Overall, this model looks good at sorting out the non-elite teams but less precise with the most successful TRUE teams. Given it is a small data set, this visual supports an acceptable model with some useful class separation.

Another way to evaluate models is with key performance indicators. There are many types of statistical evaluations related to model evaluation. Here, we cover only the basics because the point of the SEMMA workflow is not a production model rather the explanatory insights to be gained from the model. A common evaluation for a binary classification is simply accuracy. This is a measure of how often the model is correct, correctly classifying both TRUE and FALSE, among all opportunities. Accuracy is a good measure when the data is balanced, and the use applied case has an equal cost to correct TRUE and

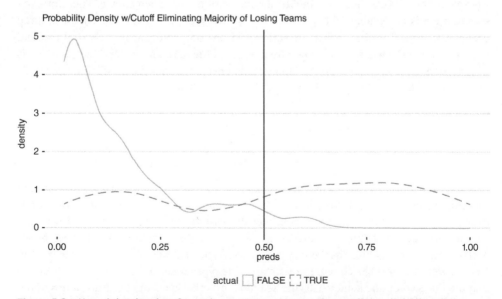

Figure 5.2 Kernel density plots for each actual team class and a cutoff threshold line that demonstrates the model's ability to separate the classes based on the training data.

correct FALSE classifications. As a result, accuracy is not always the best measure though it is common. The `MLmetrics` library has a function `Accuracy` which accepts a vector of classifications and true outcomes. The result is a number between 0 and 1 representing the overall accuracy for both success and failure classes. In this example, the result is approximately `0.88`.

```
Accuracy(y_pred = plotDF$class, y_true = plotDF$actual)
```

Creating a confusion matrix helps further understand the model behavior and can also make the accuracy measure more understandable. The following code uses `table` with the classification outcome variable, `class`, and the true outcomes in the `actual` vector. This tallies the values as shown in Table 5.3.

```
confMat <- table(plotDF$class, plotDF$actual)
```

To calculate the overall accuracy, sum the diagonal values of the matrix then divide by the overall sum of the matrix. The code below calls `sum` along with `diag` within the numerator and then simply `sum` for the entire table to obtain the same accuracy value `0.88`.

```
sum(diag(confMat))/sum(confMat)
```

One can visualize the confusion matrix's four components as an area chart with `autoplot` from the `yardstick` package. Within the function the output is a `ggplot` visual so applying a theme or title is possible by adding subsequent layers as shown.

```
autoplot(conf_mat(confMat))+
  theme_hc() +
  ggtitle('in-sample confusion matrix')
```

Another common metric in binary classification model evaluation is `LogLoss`. This metric indicates how close a probability is to the actual value. For example, conceptually it is assessing TRUE records with 0.95 probability as better than TRUE records with 0.5 probability even though both would be considered accurate. The converse is also assessed where FALSE records with low probabilities, such as 0.01, are considered better than FALSE records with 0.49 probabilities. The larger these divergences from the actual outcome, the higher the log-loss. Although it is *not* a simple measure of differences between probabilities and actuals in practice, log-loss should be minimized. Once again `MLmetrics` has a function `LogLoss` which accepts predictions and actuals. Here the value is `0.36`. While this number may be unintuitive, it will be contextualized for consistency when applied to the validation partition.

```
LogLoss(y_pred = plotDF$preds, y_true = plotDF$actual)
```

Table 5.3 The model's in-sample confusion matrix, where the intersection of the FALSE and TRUE cells represents the correctly classified teams.

	FALSE−actual	TRUE−actual
FALSE—model classification	318	35
TRUE—model classification	15	72

Table 5.4 External Kappa context from a Biochemia Medica article.

Kappa value	Level of agreement
0.0–0.20	None
0.21–0.39	Minimal
0.40–0.59	Weak
0.60–0.79	Moderate
0.80–0.90	Strong
Above 0.90	Almost perfect

Another useful matrix is the Cohen Kappa metric. This is particularly useful when you have an unbalanced data set. For example, classifying the probability of an injury can be hard because the majority of athletes do not get injured in a season. The majority class would be "non-injured" and a model could appear accurate simply by marking all records as "non-injured." However, this model would not help identify the class of interest representing the minority of injured athletes. The Cohen Kappa metric tells you how much better your model is over a random classifier that is based class frequencies.[1] The metric measures the model performance against an informed guess. To interpret this metric, values below 0 would be a model that is worse than a chance agreement with the informed guess, while a value of 1 means perfect agreement. The abridged Table 5.4 is from Biochemia Medica, an academic journal that helps contextualize the Kappa statistic.[2] In clinical psychology and medical work, a high Kappa value is required. In practice, and with a small sports related data set, a lower value is likely acceptable because the consequences are lower.

To calculate the Cohen Kappa, apply `Kappa` from `vcd`. The function accepts a confusion matrix. To review the matrix along with the confidence intervals, the `print` function is applied with an additional parameter set to `TRUE`. This model's KAPPA value is `0.67` with a lower and upper bound of `0.58` and `0.75`, respectively. When exploring data, if the value is "Minimal," one can often improve the results by adding more variables to the data set. Conceptually this brings in more information which the model can use for improved pattern recognition. According to Table 5.4, the offensive statistic shows a "moderate" amount of agreement and is a positive sign for the model's performance.

```
K <- Kappa(confMat)
print(K, CI = TRUE)
```

The next area of focus is assessing the validation set performance. Recall, the goal is to avoid over-fitting and have consistency among partitions for the model diagnostics. Revisiting the assessment workflow, construct the `validationPreds` vector using `predict` but ensure the model object is applied to the out-of-sample data in the

---

1 Jakub Czakon Mostly an ML person. Building MLOps tools, Czakon, J., Mostly an ML person. Building MLOps tools, & on, F. me. (2021, July 19). *24 evaluation metrics for binary classification (and when to use them)*. neptune.ai. https://neptune.ai/blog/evaluation-metrics-binary-classification.

2 McHugh M. L. (2012). Interrater reliability: the kappa statistic. *Biochemia Medica*, 22(3), 276–282.

`validationData` object. These probabilities are the first vector of the `valDF` data. frame. The second and third columns represent the validation set actuals, the `winning-Season` vector, and the model's classification according to the `cutoff` threshold, respectively.

```
validationPreds <- predict(fit,
                           validationData[,5:11],
                           type = 'response')
valDF <- data.frame(preds = validationPreds,
                    actual = validationData$winningSeason,
                    class = ifelse(validationPreds>=cutoff,T,F))
```

Calculating the same metrics as before is simple with the similar `valDF` data frame. The comparative results for `Accuracy`, `LogLoss`, and `Kappa` are illustrated in Table 5.5. Since the validation set represents real world outcomes since the data was not used in training, the metrics are expected to reduce slightly but not be extremely different than in-sample metrics.

```
Accuracy(y_pred = valDF$class, y_true = valDF$actual)
confMValidation <- table(valDF$class, valDF$actual)
confMValidation
LogLoss(y_pred = valDF$preds, y_true = valDF$actual)
Kval <- Kappa(confMValidation)
print(Kval, CI = TRUE)
```

The end result is a model that appears to be consistent in its understanding of basketball statistics' impact to elite and non-elite team outcomes. With this understanding the model can be examined to extract insights explaining the game statistics relationship to the outcome. Similar to linear regression, a logistic regression has beta coefficients for each informative variable. These models are said to be parametric because the coefficients represent a parameter used for prediction. This contrasts with nonparametric models like K-nearest neighbor. To review coefficient names and value, apply `coefficients` to the model object.

```
coeffs <- coefficients(fit)
coeffs
```

The coefficient values are the log-odds relationship to the outcome. To make this more intuitive, the entire range of the coefficients can be calculated, and each individual coefficient value represents a proportion of the range. Simply put, a coefficient represents some amount of the explained phenomena and the elite team outcomes, and the total

Table 5.5 A comparison of model metrics showing consistency and the expected slight decline to the validation set.

Metric	In-sample training result	Out-of-sample validation result
Accuracy	0.88	0.85
LogLoss	0.36	0.39
Kappa	0.67 (0.58–0.75)	0.57 (0.38–0.75)

absolute sum represents all the explanatory power of the model. The *y*-intercept is purposefully removed in the following code. Intuitively the *y*-intercept may represent the very essence of being a Division I Women's basketball team in terms of log-odds for elite outcomes or simply an uninformative feature of the fit model.

One can adjust the formula in the preceding `glm` fit to remove the *y*-intercept but this often impacts the model's performance. If that is necessary, append a `+0` after the period to force the intercept to 0. Since the goal of the work is explanatory power among specific statistics, the *y*-intercept is retained in model training to improve the model's pattern recognition but then removed as not germane to the overall practical effort.

The individual statistic impacts are calculated in `impact` by employing `proportions` on the absolute values of `coeffs`. The absolute `abs` function is used because the total amount of the explanatory power is under consideration and some statistics may have a negative coefficient. The square brackets index from the second variable to the end of the formula. This automatically drops the *y*-intercept since it is the first returned coefficient in the model object. Next, the floating-point numbers are sorted and then rounded to three decimal points.

```
impact <- proportions(abs(coeffs[2:length(coeffs)]))
impact <- round(sort(impact),3)
```

Although this is numeric information, the relationship among them is important. The sum of the proportionality will be 1. To the practitioner or coach, individual values are not contextualized since they represent a log-odds outcome for the success class but the interaction among attributes is noteworthy. Thus, a `waterfall` chart can help illustrate the interplay of beta proportionalities. This function accepts the proportional values and then the labels. Similar to the `autoplot` visual, the `waterfall` function employs `ggplot` so adjustments are straightforward with `theme_hc` and a `ggtitle`. Figure 5.3 is the resulting waterfall demonstrating the first interesting finding of the analysis.

```
waterfall(values = impact,
          labels = names(impact)) +
  theme_hc() +
  ggtitle('Model Attribute Proportion of Explaining Winning Teams')
```

The proportional coefficient waterfall chart shows that the `FG_PCT` accounts for nearly one-third of the model's basketball explanatory power. This may indicate that aspiring teams should focus on taking high-probability shots over other statistics like free throws and rebounds. Further, the total points per game, `PPG`, have little explanatory power leading one to believe that among Division I Women's basketball teams, taking high-probability shots is more important than the total points in a game. In fact, looking at `coeffs`, the `PPG` statistic has a slightly negative value! This means that as the points per game increases, it has a decreasing effect on being part of the success class. Still, the waterfall shows the impact is nearly nothing but contextualized with the coefficient value, `PPG` retains an ever so slightly negative influence. Instead, "clean looks" inside the three-point arc are behaviors that differentiate successful teams more so than other offensive focuses. It is not to say that rebounds or other positive coefficients are not helpful, but the model learned these efforts are less helpful than the largest waterfall area, `FG_PCT`.

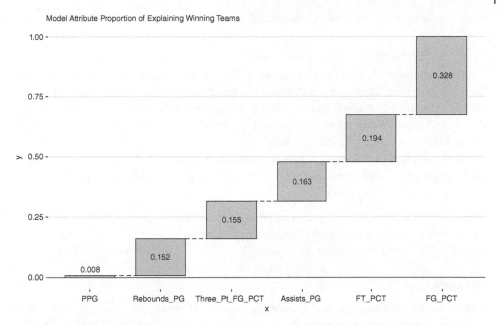

Figure 5.3 The proportional coefficient waterfall chart identifying teams with a winning percentage above the third quartile.

Table 5.6 The first six records of the winning season teams' data.

Name	Yr	Win	Loss	PPG	FG_PCT	Three_Pt_FG_PCT	FT_PCT	Rebounds_PG	Assists_PG	winning Season
Notre Dame	2014	29	5	77.3	45.4	38.7	74.9	41.7	18.2	TRUE
Nebraska	2020	32	1	77.7	46.0	38.6	77.6	39.0	16.6	TRUE
Stanford	2020	33	1	77.7	47.6	36.7	73.5	44.7	17.9	TRUE
Ohio St	2012	31	5	78.0	45.8	40.2	76.1	40.8	17.2	TRUE
Ohio St	2015	31	5	78.0	45.8	40.2	76.1	40.8	17.2	TRUE
Gonzaga	2016	29	4	80.7	47.7	37.3	73.7	41.5	19.3	TRUE

The model can likely be improved with additional statistics which affect the waterfall interpretation. Further, keep in mind this may change by division, league, or gender. The waterfall observations are only applicable to Women's Collegiate Division I basketball data. These interpretations do not generalize to all of basketball. As is the case with all machine learning models used for explanatory purposes, the insights are based narrowly on the data presented and use case.

Since the goal is to explicitly understand success, the following code uses `subset` to reduce the data when `winningSeason` equals `TRUE`. Table 5.6 is a small section of the data obtained by applying `head` to the resulting `winningTeams` object.

```
winningTeams <- subset(trainingData,
                       trainingData$winningSeason=='TRUE')
head(winningTeams)
```

In order to make a "sum-of-betas" impact by "frequency," some data munging is needed. To begin, use indexing select the statistical column `5:10`. Then for each column-wise statistic, calculate the mean average. This is performed with `apply`, then by applying the `margin` parameter where a 1 would apply functions row-wise and 2 column-wise. The last parameter is the function to be applied, here as `mean`. Next, a `data.frame` is constructed where each statistics' mean is captured as a vector. This step will create duplicative `rownames` since the result of `apply` is a named vector. Thus, the last line simply removes the duplicative information.

```
winningTeamsStats <- winningTeams[,5:10]
plotDF <- apply(winningTeamsStats,2,mean)
plotDF <- data.frame(stat              = names(plotDF),
                     avgWinningTeamValues = plotDF)
rownames(plotDF) <- NULL
```

Next, each individual statistics' impact is appended. However, the `impact` object was sorted previously so one cannot simply use `cbind` or similar. Instead within square brackets and to the left of the comma, rows are matched using `match`. The `match` function returns a vector of the position of the first parameter that corresponds to the second input. The `plotDF` data frame from the previous code is rearranged row-wise to match the existing `impact` object. Once this reorganization occurs, a new column is appended as `impact` on the left side of the assignment operator and the `impact` object on the right. This process is repeated to `match` the non-intercept coefficients with the `coeffs` object.

```
plotDF        <- plotDF[match(names(impact), plotDF$stat),]
plotDF$impact <- impact
plotDF        <- plotDF[match(names(coeffs[2:length(coeffs)]),
                              plotDF$stat),]
plotDF$coeffs <- coeffs[2:length(coeffs)]
```

Next, the upcoming plot will need to have a color-coded point since some variables have a positive sign and others a negative sign. The `ifelse` statement creates a logical condition whether or not the `coeffs` column is positive or negative and returns the quoted string `Positive` or `Negative`, respectively. Table 5.7 is the complete `plotDF` object for review which shows aspects of winning team statistics and model behavior. The table itself can be useful to practitioners because it represents aspect of winning team play which could help coaches focus efforts to improve. However, people often respond to visuals, so additional data manipulation is needed to increase the explanatory insights.

```
plotDF$coeffSign <- ifelse(plotDF$coeffs>0,'Positive','Negative')
plotDF
```

Now, the code will calculate the percent among all winning teams that have a particular statistic above the average. One cannot assume it is normally distributed even among these top teams, `for` loop is needed to explore each statistic. This frequency measure

Table 5.7 The summary winning team statistic and model data.

Stat	avgWinningTeamValues	Impact	Coeffs	coeffSign
PPG	75.79439	0.008	-0.02790597	Negative
FG_PCT	46.43551	0.328	1.17479488	Positive
Three_Pt_FG_PCT	37.28131	0.155	0.55573592	Positive
FT_PCT	75.46916	0.194	0.69312298	Positive
Rebounds_PG	42.22710	0.152	0.54591035	Positive
Assists_PG	17.08318	0.163	0.58304372	Positive

will contextualize the true elite and also how easy it is to be above average in a statistic. The code below first creates an empty vector, `tmp`, which is a temporary object to capture the calculation. Within a `for` loop, the `i` variable is iterated upon. In the `singleStat` object, a single column is selected from `winningTeamsStats`. This is performed in a square bracket index to the right of the comma. However, the `i` variable is actually nested in the `plotDF[i,1]`. For example, the first time through `i` is 1. This will select `PPG` data vector. The average value is similarly captured in the `avgStat` object where the row is still defined with `i` but corresponds to the single value in the second column. Once the `singleStat` and `avgStat` objects are defined with a particular `i` value, a simple `ifelse` operator will check whether a team's statistic, `singleStat`, is greater than or equal to the individual average, `avgStat`. The result is either a 1 or 0. Next the `teamProp` object represents the proportion of teams whose statistics is greater than average. This is calculated by summing the `1` of the preceding `ifelse` statement and dividing by the length of the `singleStat` column. This single result is captured in the `i` position of the `tmp` vector. In a sense, the vector is "filled up" as the calculation is performed for each statistic.

```
tmp <- vector()
for(i in 1:nrow(plotDF)){
  singleStat <- winningTeamsStats[,plotDF[i,1]]
  avgStat <- plotDF[i,2]
  teamCount <- ifelse(singleStat>=avgStat, 1,0)
  teamProp <- sum(teamCount) / length(singleStat)
  tmp[i] <- teamProp
  }
```

The `tmp` vector was calculated in the order of the `plotDF` object. Thus, it can be appended on the right side of the assignment while a new column is declared as `statFreq` on the left. Another column is added using `paste`. This function concatenates strings. Here the command joins the `stat` function to a string `Avg Val` and the rounded `avgWinningTeamValues` column.

```
plotDF$statFreq <- tmp
plotDF$labels <- paste(plotDF$stat,'Avg Val',round(plotDF$avgW
inningTeamValues))
```

Before constructing the visual, some additional calculations are needed to aid the audience interpretation. The upcoming code adds a vertical and horizontal line, so that the plot has quadrants. Breaking up the scatter plot into quadrants will help the audience quickly identify statistics that should be prioritized versus not. To further aid this understanding, the plot needs quadrant annotations centrally placed in each section. The annotations need x and y coordinates. The code below employs simple arithmetic to obtain x and y values. The first value, `x1`, is calculated using the `mean` of `statFreq` minus the `min` of `statFreq`. This difference is then divided by 2. Finally, this value, representing the *half-way* point from the average to the minimum, is subtracted from the overall `mean` of `statFreq`. A similar approach is employed to identify the half-way points vertically and horizontally for each of the four quadrants. The mechanics are similar but the signs change depending on the quadrant and midway point needed.

```
x1 <- mean(plotDF$statFreq) -
  ((mean(plotDF$statFreq) - min(plotDF$statFreq) ) /2)
x2 <- mean(plotDF$statFreq) +
  ((max(plotDF$statFreq) - mean(plotDF$statFreq) ) /2)
y1 <- mean(plotDF$impact) -
  ((mean(plotDF$impact) - min(plotDF$impact) ) /2)
y2 <- mean(plotDF$impact) +
  ((max(plotDF$impact) - mean(plotDF$impact) ) /2)
```

Finally, let's construct the visual that should yield some game insights. The `ggplot` plot is instantiated with `plotDF` and declares the aesthetics as `x = statFreq` and `y = impact`. The next layer adds `geom_point` while also declaring the `coeffSign` factor levels as the color labels and point shape. Additionally, the point size is adjusted so the audience can see them more readily. The point labels are added with the `geom_text` layer referring to the `stat` column. The labels are adjusted horizontally, vertically, and in size, so labels do not run off the plot itself with `hjust`, `vjust`, and `size`, respectively. Next, a vertical line is added with `geom_vline`. The intercept is the `mean` average of `statFreq` and the line is made semitransparent with the `alpha = 0.25` parameter. Similarly, a horizontal line is added with `geom_hline` referring to the `mean` of the `impact` column. To avoid visual clutter, the `theme_few` theme is appended next. Then `ggtitle` is used with an appropriate string to add a simple title. Finally, the last four layers add the `annotate` text at the predefined coordinates. Essentially, the y-axis represents basketball effort the model has determined to be important or not, by coefficient impact. The x-axis represents the percentage of teams that are above or below average compared to other winning teams. Thus, the x-axis represents the overall focus of elite teams, whether a basketball action measured in a statistic is prioritized.

```
p1 <- ggplot(plotDF, aes(x = statFreq, y = impact)) +
  geom_point(aes(color = coeffSign, shape = coeffSign)) +
  geom_text(aes(label = stat),
            size = 3.5, vjust = 1, hjust = 'inward') +
  geom_vline(aes(xintercept = mean(statFreq)), alpha = 0.25) +
  geom_hline(aes(yintercept = mean(impact)), alpha = 0.25) +
```

```
theme_few() +
ggtitle('Succesful Teams Focus Vs Model Coefficient Impact
to Winning') +
annotate("text", x = x1, y = y1,
         alpha = 0.25, label = "Unknown, Unimportant") +
annotate("text", x = x1, y = y2,
         alpha = 0.25, label = "Unknown, Important") +
annotate("text", x = x2, y = y1,
         alpha = 0.25, label = "Known, Unimportant") +
annotate("text", x = x2, y = y2,
         alpha = 0.25, label = "Known, Important")
pl
```

The object `pl` is shown in Figure 5.4. To interpret the plot, consider the quadrants and contextualize the values. In this example for Division I Women's basketball teams with winning regular seasons, the model and team frequency show that `FT_PCT` is a common and important factor among winning teams. This statistic is the only one in the upper right quadrant. Interestingly, an aspiring team could focus on `FG_PCT` over other statistics game because fewer winning teams prioritize this statistic. Statistics in the

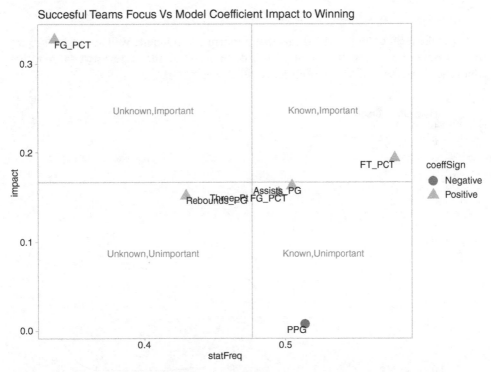

Figure 5.4 The winning team frequency by model impact regarding a winning season illustrates that free-throw percent is important yet most winning teams perform well. In contrast, the field goal percentage is important, but it is less of a focus among winning teams. This may indicate a statistic an aspiring team could focus upon to differentiate itself.

upper left quadrant may indicate a point of impactful differentiation compared to other statistics, so a team could focus on moving statistics from upper left to upper right while holding all other statistics constant. Another possible insight may be that `Rebounds_PG` have a middling winning impact and most teams do not focus on it. This is because this is the only statistic in the lower left. Collectively, coaching may have observed offensive rebounds are less helpful than free throws, assists, and three point field goal percentages. So, if a team could focus on either offensive rebounds or just field goals, the intention should be clear according to the model's output, upper left is more impactful than lower left.

Since the visual supports a focus on `FG_PCT`, let's examine it explicitly using `summary`. Next, a simple kernel density plot is called with code used previously. Of course, this visual could have been constructed during EDA but without the model's explanatory insight, the visual was not contextualized. Figure 5.5 shows a non-normal distribution of field goal percentage. As one may intuit in the previous visual, there are a small number of teams that have recognized the value of field goal percentage above other statistics.

```
summary(winningTeams$FG_PCT)
ggplot(winningTeams, aes(x = FG_PCT)) +
  geom_density() +
  theme_hc() +
  ggtitle('Field Goal Percentage')
```

Let's take a closer look at the teams that perform exceptionally well at `FG_PCT`. As a non-normal distribution, the `median` is used to `subset` the `winningTeams` rather than the mean average. The new object is called `topFGPct`.

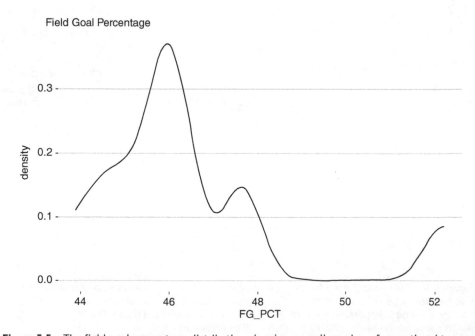

Figure 5.5 The field goal percentage distribution showing a small number of exceptional teams.

```
topFGPct <- subset(winningTeams,
                    winningTeams$FG_PCT > median(winningTeams$FG_
                    PCT))
```

In the following code, a new column is appended as `winPCT` on the left of the assignment. It is calculated as the number of team wins divided by the sum of wins and losses which represent all regular season games in a season.

```
topFGPct$winPCT <- (topFGPct$win/(topFGPct$win +
                                  topFGPct$loss))
```

Reviewing this extreme subsection of the data shows teams with a minimum winning percentage of 84.8%! Teams that perform well with this statistic, and likely others, are very successful indeed. However, the tally of the teams shown in Table 5.8 shows an unexpected 'NAME'. In Division I Women's basketball, it is often the case that Connecticut, Tennessee, Stanford, and Gonzaga are among the best.

```
summary(topFGPct$winPCT)
table(topFGPct$NAME)
```

Clearly the Green Bay women's team has found a way to differentiate itself successfully. The team likely attracts less choice athletes yet is consistently a top performer in it's respective league. One contributing factor to their success is support analytically. The data leads one to believe that Green Bay excels at field goal percentage while the model leads denote that this statistic is extremely important. In fact, according to Wikipedia,[3] the Green Bay Phoenix have been successful for some time, stating "In 2017–18, Green Bay captured its 20th straight regular season title and 16th league tournament title. The program made its 18th appearance in the NCAA Tournament, finishing the season 29–4, winning 27 games or more for the fourth consecutive year." The data and more importantly the results support their inclusion among the traditionally cited elite teams, Go Green Bay Phoenix!

Extending the Method Demonstrated

This data set is relatively limited. One can add more statistics as columns in the data set. This may dissipate the "signal" in the model across more variables making the plots have "clusters" visually but could yield multiple items to focus on or avoid depending on their respective quadrant.

Table 5.8 The inclusion of Green Bay among these traditionally elite teams is an interesting finding.

Connecticut	Gonzaga	Green Bay	Stanford	Tennessee
10	9	8	8	9

---

3 Wikimedia Foundation. (2021, March 25). *Green bay phoenix women's basketball*. Wikipedia. https://en.wikipedia.org/wiki/Green_Bay_Phoenix_women's_basketball.

Additionally, this method is not limited to basketball or women's sports. This technique can be applied any time there is a logistic regression and a need for explanation. Thus, structuring a sports problem as a binary outcome with logistic regression in other fields like Men's basketball or other sports may yield interesting insights as well.

Exercises

1) Describe the difference between explanatory and predictive modeling.

2) What is the conceptual difference between continuous classification explanatory modeling?

3) Perform the SEMMA analysis using the defensive statistics at `https://raw.githubusercontent.com/kwartler/Practical_Sports_Analytics/main/C5_Data/imputed_DefensiveStats.csv`
   a) Evaluate the model according to 'Accuracy', 'LogLoss', and 'Kappa'. Is there consistency between data partitions?

4) Create a defensive statistic waterfall chart.
   a) What is the most impactful defensive statistic proportionally? *Hint: Largest section of the waterfall.*
   b) What is the least impact defensive statistic proportionally? *Hint: Smallest section of the waterfall.*
   c) Interpret the results of the defensive proportional waterfall. *Hint: Keep in mind some defensive measures are positive basketball outcomes and others negative. Some statistics need to be evaluated along with their beta sign, positive or negative. For example,* `Opponent_Points_PG` *has a negative. This contrasts with* `Steals_PG` *which is a positive coefficient. Do not simply discount negative coefficients as basketball attributes to be ignored in favor of positive statistical measures.*

5) Create the frequency by impact scatter plot to identify areas of opportunity for aspiring teams.
   a) Identify a statistic aspiring teams should focus on. What is the sign of the coefficient? Should a team maximize or minimize this measure when playing?
   b) Review the distribution of the most impactful and overlooked statistic, and using the 'mean', identify top teams in this statistic.

6) Identify the Ivy League team among the results.
   a) Search online for any headlines citing this team for exceptional defense in 2019 or 2020 and provide a quote supporting the defensive prowess of the team. Does the model support the finding that regular season success stems from particular statistics that are modeled as important?

6

Gauging Fan Sentiment in Cricket

Objectives

- Learn what NLP is and a basic approach to analyzing text
- Learn the basic NLP terms and object classes
- Define the six-step NLP workflow
- Apply various string manipulation functions to a collection of forum posts as documents
- Identify two-word lexicons for sentiment analysis and adjust one for the forum's context
- Programmatically change the tokenization of the text from unigram to bigrams
- Learn about full, inner, and left joins
- Visualize the overall forum community comment velocity
- Build a word cloud of frequent two-word phrases
- Classify forum comments by emotional category, then plot as a radar chart for the entire forum conversation
- Focusing on individual users, calculate and visualize the network graph of comments to identify the most central author
- Individually review the most and least negative authors, creating a bar chart for review

R Libraries

```
RedditExtractoR
RCurl
lubridate
tm
qdapRegex
dplyr
echarts4r
slam
tidytext
corpus
ggplot2
ggthemes
```

```
ggwordcloud
ggradar
```

R Functions

```
get_reddit
getURL
read.csv
function
tm_map
content_transformer
rm_url
tolower
removeWords
removePunctuation
removeNumbers
stripWhitespace
c
stopwords
unlist
lapply
ngrams
words
paste
data
data.frame
rbind
dmy
year
month
day
weekdays
quarter
aggregate
sum
full_join
as.Date
cumsum
ggplot
aes
geom_area
geom_line
geom_point
ggtitle
```

```
theme_hc
%>%
e_charts
e_area
e_tooltip
e_toolbox_feature
e_theme
e_datazoom
Sys.Date()
subset
Encoding
iconv
VCorpus
VectorSource
DocumentTermMatrix
dim
col_sums
sort
rownames
head
ggwordcloud
geom_text_wordcloud_area
theme_minimal
scale_color_gradient
e_color_range
e_cloud
tidy
inner_join
str
order
round
ggradar
e_radar
get_sentiments
left_join
as.data.frame
is.na
seq_along
summary
which.min
geom_line
e_datazoom
user_network
e_graph_nodes
e_graph_edges
```

```
slice_max
slice_min
as.matrix
table
/
factor
unique
as.character
quantile
|
geom_col
scale_fill_gradient
theme
e_bar
e_visual_map
```

Sports Context

Sports marketers consistently find ways for fans to engage with the team. A team's popularity is often driven by wins but not solely by winning. In fact, teams are often asked to perform public service announcements, mascots make cameo appearances at nonsporting events, and players are encouraged to engage with fans online in social media. A data-driven sports marketer needs to measure this engagement over time to understand the marketing efforts' effectiveness. A sports marketer and team executives may want to know the fan reaction to trades, ticket promotions, key wins or losses, or any number of team actions. One way to measure fan engagement is with "social media listening." Social media listening is any software that monitors public online media mentions, sentiment, and or interactions. Often, though not always, this can take the form of text analysis on sites like Twitter and Reddit. In this chapter, you will build a social media listening tool extracting information for an Indian Premier League (IPL) team called the "Chennai Super Kings" (CSK) from the Reddit forum "Cricket." The CSK is among the most successful teams in the IPL with three championships as of 2018. Using R and social media techniques, the velocity of comments over time, their sentiment, and other interesting findings can be identified from tens of thousands of forum comments.

Technical Context

Human behavior can be complex and difficult to quantitatively analyze. This chapter reviews numeric information, employs social network analysis, but primarily focuses on natural language processing (NLP) to extract meaningful features from text such as common two-word phrases and sentiment analysis. Although NLP can use sophisticated machine learning techniques such as unsupervised learning and document classification, this chapter components employing NLP focus on a bag-of-words style of analysis. Bag-of-words NLP techniques use word frequency and choice rather than part of speech, word order, or abstractive meanings found in deep neural nets. This is because entire books are written on sophisticated NLP yet are outside the scope of this sports focused book. In this chapter, bag-of-words NLP follows a predictable pattern where one identifies a problem statement, organizes text, extracts features, builds visualizations, and helps the audience reach a conclusion. In the book *Text Mining in Practice with R*, six NLP project steps are outlined. These steps are described in Table 6.1 according to the CSK data.

1. **Define the problem:** The following code represents an exploratory analysis for the CSK and IPL fans.
2. **Identify the text to be collected:** The data were provided by Reddit's application program interfaces (API) searching for the "CSK" acronym on the "Cricket" subreddit found here: https://www.reddit.com/r/Cricket

As part of the text channel identification, it is important to research the nuances of the word usage. This is because lexical diversity is heavily impacted by many factors. For example, legal documents like athlete contracts will have a specific set of terms while social media or forum authors will use an altogether different set of terms. Thus, this step also encompasses research and understanding to inform the analysis.

3. **Organize the text:** The text will be organized into various data forms. In a bag-of-words NLP analysis, the primary data object is a document term matrix (DTM) described below.
4. **Extract features:** Many features will be extracted including:
   a. The number of comments over time
   b. Common two-word phrases in the forum
   c. The emotions identified
   d. The positive and negative language used over time
   e. The top 50 positive and negative authors driving the overall polarity of comments
   f. The comment authors that are central to the discussions.
5. **Analyze:** From these extracted data objects, multiple visualizations will be constructed for easy pattern recognition and audience understanding.
6. **Reach an insight:** The visuals will guide a sports marketer or other interested party to understand the velocity of the comments for the CSK, the emotional and polarized language used in comments.

NLP-specific Terms

As a niche field of data science, NLP has its own data types and definitions. As the code descriptions describe, the analysis in this chapter refer to these terms in order to ensure you are internalizing their meaning and information.

Corpus: A collection of documents for analysis.

Stopwords: High frequency with low informational value that are usually removed.

Lexicon: A collection of terms, a word list.

Token: A term or multiple terms for analysis.

Tokenization: The act of segmenting term(s) into tokens for analysis.

Polarity: The measure of the positivity or negativity of an author.

Sentiment analysis: The classification of an emotional state of an author.

Plutchik's wheel: A framework for basic emotional states theorized by psychologist Robert Plutchik.

Document term matrix: A large matrix where rows represent individual documents of a corpus and columns are unique tokens either one or more words.

Word frequency matrix: A matrix of unique terms and associated frequencies.

Ngram: The number of individual terms defined in tokenization.

Bigram: A common ngram tokenization type referring to two-word combinations in a document term matrix.

Syntactic parsing versus bag of words: This chapter demonstrates a bag-of-words analysis where word order and part of speech do not matter; this contrasts with "syntactic parsing" where the term, along with meta-information such as the part of speech, informs the analysis and methods.

Code

After loading the libraries listed above, obtain the data in one of two manners. If you prefer to work with contemporary data, use the `get_reddit` function as shown below to call the Reddit API. If you prefer to have the same data set exemplified in this chapter, download `'commentsReddit_Feb_15_2021.csv'` and use `read.csv`:

```
commentDF <- get_reddit(search_terms = 'CSK',
                        subreddit = "Cricket")
commentDF <- read.csv('commentsReddit_Feb_15_2021.csv')
```

The `commentDF` data has approximately 11,000 rows returned from the Reddit API. In this chapter, the primary data of interest is the `$comment` and `$user` columns though the data column will also be used due to the temporal nature of the forum.

Before the analysis begins, it is often a good idea to write custom functions. As the analysis gets more complex, custom functions help ensure the code is more concise and less error prone. Although this is a simple example, if you were examining two or more teams, copy and pasting code and then updating object types makes code updates more challenging, and if you miss updating an object variable, your analysis will be flawed. Thus, custom functions and even R packages can aid you!

This custom function is called `cleanCorpus` and it performs string manipulation on a corpus object. Obviously, it accepts a corpus object but also accepts stop words. Recall that stop words are high-frequency terms that yield little to no informational value. In a sense they are clutter, used by people to facilitate communication. Once these are passed into the function, the `tm_map` function maps a specific string manipulation function to the entire corpus. The majority of these functions come from the `tm` library. For functions that are not from the `tm` package, an additional function `content_trans-former` is used to nest the string manipulating function. For example, base R's `tolower` is nested in `content_transformer` which is then passed to `tm_map`. Specifically, the `cleanCorpus` function will remove URLs from the Reddit comments with the convenance function `rm_url` though it can be done with regular expressions. Next the corpus text is made lowercase as described earlier. Finally, the common `tm` package functions `removeWords`, which requires a vector of terms to remove, `removePunctuation`, `removeNumbers`, and `stripWhitespace` are applied accomplishing their respective tasks. The goal of a bag-of-words analysis is to unify terms and count their frequencies. As a result, these string manipulation steps aid term aggregation. Of course, these design choices do affect analytical outcomes. Thus, care should be taken, and iterative exploration is key to creating a trustworthy NLP analysis.

```
cleanCorpus<-function(corpus, customStopwords){
    corpus <- tm_map(corpus, content_transformer(qdapRegex::rm_url))
    corpus <- tm_map(corpus, content_transformer(tolower))
    corpus <- tm_map(corpus, removeWords, customStopwords)
    corpus <- tm_map(corpus, removePunctuation)
    corpus <- tm_map(corpus, removeNumbers)
    corpus <- tm_map(corpus, stripWhitespace)
    return(corpus)
}
```

Although the code is not being applied to the data yet, the stop words need to be determined. A simple vector called `stops` is created using an academic lexicon, "SMART," made of more than 570 common terms such as "he," "she," "the," and "it." These are combined with the `c` function to common project-specific terms. Although "cricket" is not a common stop word, in the context of a Reddit forum discussing cricket, the term is highly frequent yet contains little informational value. Similarly, the API search query was for CSK. Thus, it should be removed as highly frequent and expected. Notice the terms are lowercase in the stop words vector. In the preceding `cleanCorpus` function, `tolower` is applied *before* `removeWords`.

```
# Create custom stop words
stops <- c(tm::stopwords('SMART'), 'cricket', 'chennai', 'super',
'kings', 'csk', 'match')
```

The following analysis will use unigram, single word tokens and bi-gram, two-word tokens to construct various plots. The default DTM behavior is to create unigrams from the text. However, bigrams are often preferred for frequency analysis because it may add more context. For example, the token "bad" has a different contextual understanding than the bigram token "not bad" which includes the negation. To create n-gram tokenizations, the custom `nTokenization` function is created accepting a string document as `x` and the number of tokens to split as `n`. It will be used as a control parameter when creating the DTM. This function has a lot of functions working in concert. At the highest level, the `ngram` function is applied to the corpus list using `lapply`. The `ngram` function needs the splicing parameter to capture the number of single terms to be captured together. This output is passed to `paste` with another parameter `collapse` so that the n-gram tokens are organized. Since the entire operation occurs based on `lapply`, the output must be delivered to `unlist` so that the tokens are returned to a simple vector. If you prefer to use more than two terms per token, simply change the default function behavior `n=2` to another integer.

```
nTokenization <-function(x, n=2){
   unlist(lapply(NLP::ngrams(words(x), n), paste, collapse = " "),
         use.names = FALSE)
}
```

Although not a custom function, this analysis will utilize a public lexicon called `affect_wordnet` lexicon for analysis. This data set is shared under a Create Commons Attribution 3.0 Unported License. The `affect_wordnet`[1] is shared within the `corpus` package but is easily found online. There are multiple other lexicons such as the NRC, AFINN, or Bing lexicons which can be found within the `corpus` or `tidytext` packages. However, the `affect_wordnet` has a useful license and had terms according to their emotional affiliation. As channels, topics and needs change the corresponding lexicons will need to be adjusted. Additionally, there are third part API services or deep neural network approaches to labeling passages by sentiment. These techniques are beyond the scope of a sports-focused book as opposed to an advanced NLP book. Table 6.1 is an abridged version of the `affect_wordnet`.

Communication theory dictates that channel, messenger, and audience affect word choice. In this example, the channel is an online forum. This likely means slang terms occur and may include terms with specific meanings for the particularly subreddit. For further context, the messenger is the post author while the audience are other forum

Table 6.1 A portion of the 1641 wordnet_affect lexicon.

Term	Pos	Category	Emotion
Kid	VERB	Joy	Positive
Merry	ADJ	Joy	Positive
Anticipant	ADJ	Expectation	Ambiguous
Anxious	ADJ	Fear	Negative

---

1 Strapparava, C. and Valitutti A. (2004). WordNet-Affect: an affective extension of WordNet. *Proceedings of the 4th International Conference on Language Resources and Evaluation*, 1083–1086.

readers. As a popular sport in India with reference specific to an IPL team, it is likely the forum contains slang specific to the culture and context. To adjust a lexicon, simply create a customized lexicons specific to the channel, messenger, or audience context as part of the second step, "**Identify the text to be collected**" in the text-mining process. The `data.frame` function call below will be used to add two slang terms which have been mentioned as used within India. For example, the phrase "she belted me" corresponds to being scolded and "don't take tension" parallels "don't be stressed." Here, an object with the same columns as `affect_wordnet` is constructed. This is the customized lexicon which will be appended to the basic lexicon and can be further expanded based on more research. Table 6.2 shows the result of the code.

```
slangTerms <- data.frame(term = c('tension', 'belt'),
                    pos = c('NOUN', 'VERB'),
               category = c('Pensiveness', 'Shame'),
                emotion = c('Negative', 'Negative'))
```

The customized lexicon is easily appended to `affect_wordnet` using `rbind` as shown below.

```
affect_wordnet <- rbind(affect_wordnet, slangTerms)
```

An interesting aspect of this analysis is the temporal nature of the comments. The number of comments and emotions will fluctuate over time. As a result, multiple new data attributes can be engineered from the `post_date` column. To begin this process, apply the `lubridate` function `dmy` to the raw date column. Base-R may interpret this column as character strings of factors. The `dmy` function will transform these object types to a date class if the organization is recognized such as days, months, and years separated by dashes or slashes. Once the vector is a `Date` class, the following code extracts `year`, `month`, `day`, `weekdays`, and `quarter` using the corresponding functions. New columns are assigned to each on the left of the assignment operator. Lastly, although the book usually employs the camel-case code style (i.e., camelCase), for consistency with the original data frame, the new columns are separated with underscores (i.e., post_date_yr).

```
commentDF$post_date <- dmy(commentDF$post_date)
commentDF$post_date_yr <- year(commentDF$post_date)
commentDF$post_date_month <- month(commentDF$post_date)
commentDF$post_date_day <- day(commentDF$post_date)
commentDF$post_date_weekday <- weekdays(commentDF$post_date)
commentDF$post_date_weekday <- quarter(commentDF$post_date)
```

Table 6.2 The small, customized lexicon for context specific emotional slang terms.

Term	Pos	Category	Emotion
tension	NOUN	Pensiveness	Negative
belt	VERB	Shame	Negative

The same approach can be applied to the comment date. The data is separated because a forum post may occur on 1 day with follow-up comments occurring on the same, subsequent day or even across multiple days. Although only some of these engineered variables are used for visualizations in this chapter, one can explore the various other temporal meta-data by simply adjusting the example code to these other attributes like month or quarter.

```
commentDF$comm_date <- dmy(commentDF$comm_date)
commentDF$comm_date_yr <- year(commentDF$comm_date)
commentDF$comm_date_month <- month(commentDF$comm_date)
commentDF$comm_date_day <- day(commentDF$comm_date)
commentDF$comm_date_weekday <- weekdays(commentDF$comm_date)
commentDF$comm_date_weekday <- quarter(commentDF$comm_date)
```

An interesting aspect of the forum is the velocity, meaning the number of new posts or comments over time. This can be done by assigning a value of `1` for each row, then employing `aggregate`. The `aggregate` function accepts a formula defining the aggregation of the data and a function to be applied. Here, the new count column, `ct` with a value of `1`, is aggregated by the `comm_date` column where `sum` is applied to each comment date. Similarly, the `aggregate` function is applied to the `post_date` by adjusting the function. One can add more aggregation columns such as `ct ~ post_date + title` which will aggregate the `ct` column by post-date and the title before applying `sum`. This is done for example only in the following code. Then, the `title` column is deleted with `NULL` because this information is not actually needed.

```
commentDF$ct <- 1
commSum <- aggregate(ct~comm_date, commentDF, sum)
postSum <- aggregate(ct~post_date + title, commentDF, sum)
postSum$title <- NULL
```

Next, the two data objects are merged using a `full_join`. Figure 6.1 conceptually illustrates a "full join" where all data is retained between two tables. In this data, when dates are shared, the columns are appended, and when a date only has one feature such as only a post with no comments, an `NA` is filled in.

```
areaChart <- full_join(commSum,
                       postSum,
                       by = c('comm_date'='post_date'))
```

The result of the join needs improved naming to ensure the analysis is error free. Thus, the `names` function is applied on the left of the assignment operator along with a corresponding vector of common-sense column names. Keep in mind the order of the tables needs account for the conforming column names. Care must be taken to not mislabel the joined data.

```
names(areaChart) <- c('dates','newComments','newPosts')
```

Although not actually the case here, data manipulation may coerce a "Date" column to an unordered factor. To ensure the visual is constructed temporally, the following code

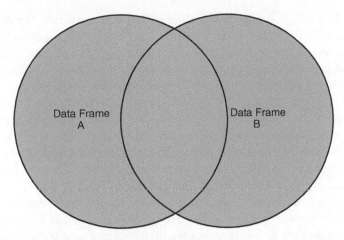

Figure 6.1 A full join where all data in table A is appended to table B and NAs are used to fill in non-shared key value pairs.

reapplies `as.Date` to the `dates` column within the `order` function. In this specific example, the format is declared as `format="%Y/%M/%D"`. These nested functions appear on the left of the data frames comma. The column is confirmed to be a "Date" object type, then ordered by time and that affected the entire data frame `areaChart`. Since the default behavior of `full_join` is to fill in with `NA`, the entire data frame will be searched for NA with `is.na` and, if identified, is declared as 0.

```
areaChart <- areaChart[order(as.Date(areaChart$dates,
                                format="%Y/%M/%D")),]
areaChart[is.na(areaChart)] <- 0
```

Finally, the cumulative sum function `cumsum` is applied to the `newComments` and `newPosts` columns to create new features. A cumulative sum is a running total of a vector of terms. For example, a cumulative sum of a vector including 1, 3, and 5 would result in 1, 4 (3 + 1) and 9 (4 + 5). Table 6.3 shows the results of the aggregation, NA to 0 and construction of cumulative sum columns for the first four dates.

```
areaChart$cumulativeComments <- cumsum(areaChart$newComments)
areaChart$cumulativePosts <- cumsum(areaChart$newPosts)
```

Using this data frame, construct a static image with `ggplot2` and `ggthemes`. First, a best practice is to create a chart title string as the variable `chartTitle`. Next instantiate

Table 6.3 A portion of the comments and posts by day.

Dates	newComments	newPosts	cumulativeComments	cumulativePosts
2014-02-12	450	478	450	478
2014-02-13	28	0	478	478
2014-05-30	288	291	766	769
2014-05-31	3	0	769	769

the visual with `ggplot` passing in the data and declaring aesthetics. The *x*-axis refers to the `dates` column while the *y*-axis refers to the `cumulativeComments`. The next layer adds the area plot with `geom_area` filled with an explicit hex color code. A color hex code represents red, green, and blue color mixtures explicitly, so colors are consistent. The alpha parameter adds some transparency to the colored area of the chart. The next layer adds a line on top of the semi-transparent area with `geom_line` along with a `0.5` thickness and slightly darker color. Yet, another layer is added for specific points using `geom_point`. The size of the dot is declared along with a coordinated color. The end effect is a pleasing area chart punctuated by the specific points that are connected temporally as a line chart. The last two layers add the title and apply a preconstructed High Charts style chart. Figure 6.2 is the result of the various `ggplot` function called showing a dramatic increase in comment velocity more recently in the forum. Often in these types of analyses, an intensification of post or comment velocity is triggered by an event, such as a controversial post, athlete behavior, key win or loss, or significant personnel change made by a team.

```
chartTitle <- 'Cumulative Comments Over Time'
ggplot(areaChart, aes(x=dates, y=cumulativeComments))+
    geom_area(fill="#bada55", alpha=0.4) +
    geom_line(color="#02AC1E", size=0.5) +
    geom_point(size=1, color="#02AC1E") +
    ggtitle(chartTitle) + theme_hc()
```

It may be more useful for a user to zoom into the dates, particularly if there are more points that begin to crowd the plot day to day. A JavaScript enabled web visual can accomplish this within the `echarts4r` package. To make an interactive plot, the `areaChart` data is forwarded to the `e_charts` plot instantiation function. Within `e_charts`, the

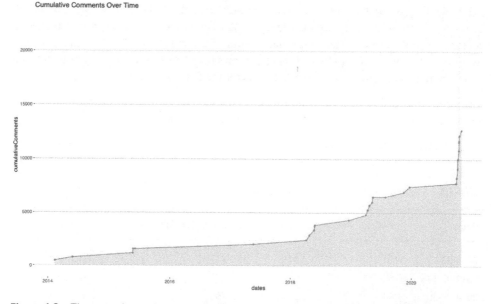

Figure 6.2 The area chart with dramatically increasing comment velocity in recent dates.

`dates` column declares the *x*-axis. This is forwarded to `e_area` where the *y*-axis is determined as `cumulativeComments`. Functionality for the user is added with `e_tooltip`. An optional trigger type is passed as `axis` so that a user's mouse tooltip will display a points value along with a vertical dotted line. The next layer adds a "saveAsImage" ability so a user can download a static image from the dynamic plot. Overall, the colors are defined for publications with `e_theme`'s "gray" palette. Lastly, a user input "slider" is appended with `e_datazoom` which allows the user to interact and zoom into the area plot by limiting dates along the *x*-axis. Later in this chapter, the data is subset to the 2020 dates particularly to understand the sentiment. It is often useful to compare the comment vocality with the sentiment over time, shown later, but care is needed to ensure the dates are consistent between the charts.

```
areaChart %>%
  e_charts(dates) %>%
  e_area(cumulativeComments) %>%
  e_tooltip(trigger = "axis") %>%
  e_toolbox_feature(feature = "saveAsImage") %>%
  e_theme('gray') %>% e_datazoom(type = "slider")
```

An interesting aspect of language is term frequency. This can be a crude yet useful way to extract topics from a large corpus. Further, audiences often respond well to "word clouds" where individual terms are sized according to their frequency compared to a simple bar chart of term frequency. This chapter has two methods for subsetting the comment data frame. There are times that the word frequency is determined by the most frequent posts. The most recent comments can be programmatically defined or explicitly declared. First, the `Sys.date` function will update each day for the R environment. This is then differenced with 365 days. This has the effect identifying the `comm_date` 1 year ago from any `Sys.date`. No matter when the code is executed, the `idx` object will only retain all rows up to 1 year prior to that day. This is used in conjunction with the greater than sign, so a logical evaluation occurs and a vector of Boolean values is created for `idx`. One could easily change the 365 to any number of prior days to suit the analysis. Once the indexing Boolean vector is created, it is used with single brackets on the `comment` column of text.

```
idx <- commentDF$comm_date>(Sys.Date()-365)
lastYrComments <- commentDF$comment[idx]
```

Another option is to use `subset` by checking any of the engineered meta-data columns. In this code chunk, `subset` is applied only to the `comment` column. The logical condition is to check whether an engineered column `post_date_yr` is equal to `2020`. Of course, this logical condition can be adjusted to any temporal variable such as quarter or even other specific data elements. The drawback of a manually defined check is that the code needs to be updated when a new year passes, and more comments are downloaded from the Reddit API. This contrasts to the use of `Sys.date` previously illustrated.

```
lastYrComments <- subset(commentDF$comment,
               commentDF$post_date_yr==2020)
```

Sometimes text may be of mixed languages, or likely to have emojis which may not be parsed correctly within R. This may make the word cloud distracting because unknown characters may be assigned a seemingly random universal text encoding string such as U+20AC which corresponds to the special character €. In fact, this code is part of "Unicode Transformation Format" which helps computers pass and interpret characters universally. To check a character vector, apply the `Encoding` function. If the response is "unknown," this indicates R may have some trouble reading characters correctly given your local R environment settings. One method to address this is by first setting the encoding using `Encoding` with a string for the expected text type, here it is "UTF-8." This function facilitates a conversion from one text encoding to another. Once that is performed, employ `iconv` on the text vector along with parameters `from` and `to`. The last parameter is the `sub` input. If a character is a nonconvertible character byte, an NA will be added. However, in a word frequency plot, this may inflate the term occurrence of NA as a word in the comments. Thus, the `sub` parameter is set to an empty string in quotes. Although the text vector may still be "unknown" after these steps, the two functions will still impact the character strings and will improve results in many cases, especially with language not associated to your R environment.

```
Encoding(lastYrComments)
Encoding(lastYrComments) <- "UTF-8"
lastYrComments <-iconv(lastYrComments,
                    from = "UTF-8",
                    to = "ASCII",
                    sub = "")
```

Next the text needs to be preprocessed. Within a bag-of-words natural language analysis, the goal is to unify terms and then count their frequency or other weighting. As a result, text processing, basically string manipulation, is applied to unify terms. For example, the terms "CUP," "Cup," and "cup" are unified to a single token representing the information "cup." There are more complex techniques to improve term unification, most common is lemmatization or word stemming and completion, but this single chapter will focus on the foundational string manipulations often employed.

To begin the text vector needs to be declared as a `VectorSource`, so that each element of the vector is a standalone document to be processed. This is nested in the `VCorpus` function which declares the object as a corpus object. This object class is specific to the `tm` package and is a list object with documents as elements. Other document sources like `DataframeSource` can even capture document level meta-data like timestamps and authors. However, the `VectorSource` function only retains the documents themselves for the corpus. The `V` of `VCorpus` stands for volatile. This means the corpus is held in active memory. If your computer were to unexpectedly shut down, the corpus would be lost because it is held in RAM.

```
lastYrCorpus <- VCorpus(VectorSource(lastYrComments))
```

Once the data is a corpus class object, the customized `cleanCorpus` function can be applied. As previously described this function will make a series of adjustments to the raw text to unify the terms. Not only are the internal `cleanCorpus` functions customizable for the specific analysis but also the `customStopwords` parameter is customizable too. Adjusting both is part of the "art and science" of NLP making these types of analyses highly iterative. The need for additional iteration and qualitative changes particularly to the stop words may seem unscientific but understand that unlike many typical quantitative analyses, language is a humanistic and evolving affair. The terms of expression vary by person, by context, and over time. Thus, think of adjustments more as tuning parameters to the workflow than a biasing of the analysis.

```
lastYrCorpus <- cleanCorpus(lastYrCorpus, stops)
```

Depending on the length of documents or number of documents, the `cleanCorpus` may take some time to complete. When finished and the `lastYrCorpus` is called in the R console, it will be printed as a `<<VCorpus>>` with a document count corresponding to the length of the original character vector `lastYrComments`. The next step is to organize the data into a `Document Term Matrix (DTM)`. The DTM organizes the data without regard for part of speech or word order within a document. This gives rise to the name "bag of words" because the terms are jumbled within a "bag" or document. As described earlier, the `DocumentTermMatrix` function will arrange the data so that documents are rows and unique word tokens are columns. The default behavior is to count the word frequency for values and fill in 0 for any tokens not in a particular document. In the code below, the second parameter employs a `control` or instruction when constructing the DTM. This parameter employs the custom `nTokenization` function defined previously. Without this optional control, the `DocumentTermMatrix` function will create unigrams as columns. With this parameter which employs `n=2` in the custom function, the columns will be unique two-word pairs. When calling `dim` on this object, the number of rows corresponds to the number of documents and length of the original vector. The columns represent the total number of unique two-word combinations among *all* of the documents.

```
lastYrBigramDTM <- DocumentTermMatrix(lastYrCorpus,

control=list(tokenize=nTokenization))
dim(lastYrBigramDTM)
```

As expected, this is a sparse matrix with many 0s. The `lastYrBigramDTM` object is technically a "simple triplet matrix" for efficient memory use rather than a typical matrix which is less efficient. One can apply `as.matrix` from base-R to convert it to a normal matrix object type or employ functions from the `slam` package to perform matrix operations. Here, the `col_sums` function from `slam` is applied so that the object is still lightweight in memory. Otherwise, the use of base-R `as.matrix` and `colSums` can have the same result. As a NLP analysis may have many thousands, or even millions of documents, using `slam`'s functions without conversion are preferred.

```
wfm <- col_sums(lastYrBigramDTM)
```

This creates a word frequency matrix. More specifically, the `wfm` object is a bi-gram token frequency named vector. As a frequentist analysis, the `sort` function can be applied to reorder from decreasing to increasing bi-gram token usage. For simplicity, the result is organized into a two-column data frame of terms and related frequency. The

Table 6.4 A portion of the bigram frequency data frame.

Word	Freq.
Middle order	52
Strike rate	33
World cup	24
Sam curran	20
Mega auction	17
Middle overs	17

last line drops `rownames` as attributes because it is duplicative to the `word` column. Table 6.4 is a portion of the word frequency matrix to illustrate the results of the column sum on the DTM.

```
wfm <- sort(wfm, decreasing = T)
wfm <- data.frame(word = names(wfm), freq = wfm)
rownames(wfm) <- NULL
head(wfm)
```

Although this tabular data could be visualized in a bar chat, audiences relate well to word clouds. On one hand, word clouds are overused and no more informative than a bar chart, but on the other, there is no denying audiences respond to the visual type. In a word cloud, tokens are placed in an oval or circular shape. The individual terms are sized according to their associated frequency. There are multiple packages supporting word clouds such as `wordcloud` and `wordcloud2`. For consistency with other examples, a `ggplot` style package called `ggwordcloud` will be used instead. Similar to the `qplot` function, a word cloud can quickly be constructed with a single `ggwordcloud` function call. The inputs are the terms to be displayed and then the associated frequencies. These columns are only declared as rows `[1:50,]` so the visual is constructed without over-plotting. The last parameter simply adds some colors to the visual.

```
ggwordcloud(wfm[1:50, 1],
            wfm[1:50, 2],
            colors = c('grey', 'tomato'))
```

If more aesthetic control is needed, then a traditional `ggplot` layering can be used. In this example, the `ggplot` is instantiated with the first 50 rows. The aesthetics are defined with the `word` column for labels, while both size and color will refer to the `freq` column. The next layer adds the tag cloud with `geom_text_wordcloud_area`. The optional `shape` parameter has prebuilt shapes including "circle," "cardiod" (heart shaped), "diamond," "square," "triangle-forward," "triangle-upright," "pentagon," and "star." Next, the `theme_minimal` removes the typical gray background that defaults in `ggplot`. If a custom shape is needed, the package provides the ability to create a mask which acts as a silhouette which is then filled in with the tokens. However, most often a generic shape is acceptable for most audiences. The last layer creates a color scales for low-to-high values. These inputs can be named colors as shown here or can be

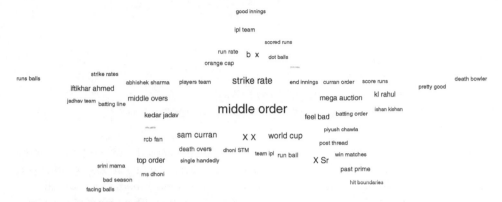

Figure 6.3 The star-shaped word cloud showing "middle order" as the most frequent token.

hexadecimal codes. Figure 6.3 is the result of the `ggwordcloud` plot. This visualizes the fact that the most used two-word combination in the forum includes "middle order" and "strike order" which may indicate popular topics among fans.

```
ggplot(wfm[1:50, ],
        aes(label = word,
            size = freq,
            color = freq))+
    geom_text_wordcloud_area(shape = 'star') +
    theme_minimal() +
    scale_color_gradient(low = "darkgrey", high = "tomato")
```

An issue with a static image word cloud is that the actual values are not known. Size is simply scaled according to the plot size so explicit values are not illustrated. Once again, `echarts4r` can provide tooltips which alert a user to the specific values. In the following code chunk, the `wfm` first 50 rows are forwarded to the `e_color_range` function. This is done before instantiating the JavaScript plot. This function accepts the data frame, and a named output column along with a color range. `e_color_range` will append a column named as the output column, `colorColumn` that scales according to the frequency values between the colors from low to high. The revised data frame is forwarded to `e_charts` to declare the plot. The `e_cloud` layer is added declaring the columns of terms, frequencies, and associated colors, respectively. The third input `colorColumn` was appended column name from `e_color_range`. Once again there is a parameter for declaring a premade shape and finally a size scale is added within `e_cloud`. Sometimes determining the `sizeRange` values it iterative depending on the number of terms in the word frequency matrix. Lastly, additional user functionality for image download and the tooltip are appended with `e_toolbox_feature` and `e_tooltip`.

```
wfm[1:50, ] %>%
    e_color_range(freq, colorColumn, colors = c("darkgrey",
"tomato")) %>%
```

```
e_charts() %>%
e_cloud(word,
        freq,
        colorColumn,
        shape = "star",
        sizeRange = c(10, 25)) %>%
e_toolbox_feature(feature = "saveAsImage") %>%
e_tooltip()
```

At this point in the analysis, the posting velocity is understood and the topics can be assumed to be "middle order," "strike rate," and "sam curran" among others. Another perspective worth exploring is the sentiment of the posts. A simple method to ascertain the emotional sentiment of authors is by performing an inner join with an emotional lexicon. A new DTM must be constructed with unigrams because the terms of the lexicon are single tokens. Thus, one must reapply `DocumentTermMatrix` without the control parameter.

```
lastYrDTM <- DocumentTermMatrix(lastYrCorpus)
```

In contrast to a wide data format like a matrix full of zeros, the inner join must be performed with a long format "tidy" object. A tidy object can be memory efficient because only key value pairs and the term frequency are retained. Its real benefit is that the data is always consistently formatted for use in other functions in the "tidy-verse" set of packages. In contrast, a traditional DTM will have term frequency and all term occurrences, with 0s and values greater than 0. The tidy format essentially throws out the 0s. To tidy a DTM, simply apply `tidy`. The following code creates the tidy version of the unigram DTM and then explores its dimensionality in comparison to the original DTM. Table 6.5 is a portion of the tidy data object with the same information as the DTM though different dimensionality.

```
lastYrTidy <- tidy(lastYrDTM)
dim(lastYrDTM)
dim(lastYrTidy)
head(lastYrTidy, 12)
```

Table 6.5 A portion of the tidy unigram data from cricket forum posts

Document	Term	Count
1	bumrah	2
1	crores	2
1	Jadhav	3
1	kedar	1
1	kick	1
1	overpaid	1
1	paid	2

Once the data is in a tidy format, an `inner_join` is performed to identify the terms in the column `leastYrTidy$term` represented in Table 6.5 that are shared with the "term" column within the `affect_wordnet` lexicon exemplified in Table 6.1. An inner join finds the intersection of data between two tables and throws out all other rows not shared. Along with the two tables, the `inner_join` column requires one or more shared column defined in the `by` parameter. Figure 6.4 is a conceptual representation of an inner join. The shaded area represents the data that is retained during the join.

```
affectSent <- inner_join(lastYrTidy,
                         affect_wordnet,
                         by=c('term' = 'term'))
```

The result of the join captured in `affectSent` retains the `document`, `term`, and `count` data and appends the `pos` (part of speech), `category`, and `emotion` from the lexicon. Calling `str` and `dim` on this joined object demonstrates the data frame structure and that lexicon matches occurred 1792 among all the documents. Keep in mind document meta-data like username and more specific timestamp could also be joined by the document number which corresponds to the original `commentDF` data frame. This emotional data corresponds broadly to the most recent year based on the `subset` performed earlier. To construct a multidimensional plot of values, the data can be aggregated. Using `aggregate` the code below performs a `sum` of the `count` column values by the emotional `category` column. Table 6.6 is result of the emotional aggregation.

```
str(affectSent)
dim(affectSent)
emos <- aggregate(count ~ category, affectSent, sum)
```

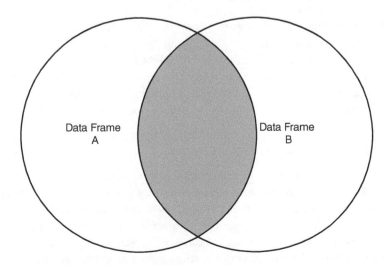

Figure 6.4 An inner join between two tables.

Table 6.6 The count and grouping of emotional words identified within all forum posts.

Category	Count
Joy	152
Love	325
Affection	102
Liking	58
Enthusiasm	70
Gratitude	1
Pride	8
Levity	1
Calmness	103
Fearlessness	32
Expectation	178
Hope	141
Sadness	250
Dislike	179
Shame	46
Compassion	11
Despair	26
Anxiety	57
Daze	8
Surprise	13
Agitation	20
Pensiveness	3

One can plot the data with all dimensions or remove low-frequency emotions to remove clutter. The following code reorders the data frame by emotional frequency in ascending order. After `order` is applied within the square brackets, the `tail` function obtains the last 10 rows when instantiating the radar chart. This ensures only the top 10 most frequent emotional categories are visualized. However, this is all optional and the radar chart can be constructed with the `emos` data frame directly by using that object instead of `emosSmall`.

```
emos <- emos[order(emos$count, decreasing = F),]
emosSmall <- tail(emos, 10)
```

Oddly, the `ggradar` package documentation does not employ data in a long format. As a result, some data manipulation is needed to ready the information. Here, a temporary data frame with one column is constructed called `tmp`. It is the result of the original `emosSmall`'s second `count` column being transposed to a wide format with `t`. Next, the `proportions` of each value are calculated. This represents the emotion category proportionally across all documents in the corpus. So, one could say "4% of the forum posts mentioning CSK show enthusiasm." Next, the column names of the `tmp` data frame are declared referring to the original `category` column. Finally, this temporary wide form object is passed to `ggradar`. Within `ggradar` the `grid.max` column determines the outermost ring value. Since all values are proportional, setting the value to `1` is appropriate. Figure 6.5 is a `ggplot` style radar chart from the code below.

```
tmp <- data.frame(t(emosSmall[,2]))
tmp <- round(proportions(tmp),2)
names(tmp) <- emosSmall$category
ggradar(tmp, grid.max = 1)
```

A more interactive and useful plot can be employed with `echarts4r`. To instantiate the plot pass either `emos` or `emosSmall` to the `e_charts` function defining `category` as the plot axes. This is forwarded to the `e_radar` layer specifying the `count` column as the value for each axes. Further, the maximum extension of the axes is defined as the `max` value of the column plus an arbitrary integer. This parameter improves aesthetics so that the chart lines and dots do not extend exactly to the outermost ring of the radar chart. Optionally, the plot values in the tooltip are renamed to "emotions." As shown previously, the `e_theme` sets the palette for publication while `e_toolbox_feature` and `e_tooltip` provide additional user interfaces.

```
emosSmall %>%
  e_charts(category) %>%
  e_radar(count,
          max = max(emos$count)+10,
          name = "emotions") %>%
  e_theme('gray') %>%
  e_toolbox_feature(feature = "saveAsImage") %>%
  e_tooltip(trigger = 'item')
```

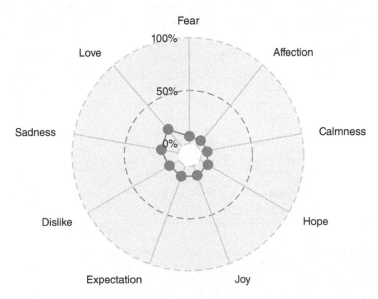

Figure 6.5 The ggplot style radar chart, showing more love terms as a proportion of the text.

Another method to assess emotional intensity in a document collection is with the `AFINN`[2] lexicon. This lexicon comes from research where 2467 terms were identified as having an emotional context, but the terms are not categorized by emotion. Instead, the words are scored on a range from +5 to −5 without 0. Rather than a specific emotional state, this is referred to as a polarity score because the terms asses positive or negative sentiment. The `tidytext` library provides the `get_sentiments` function to load a number of popular lexicons including AFINN. AFINN is shared under the "Open Database License" meaning it is free to share, create, or adapt as long as there is proper attribution, and any derivative works require open access and a similar license. Once obtained a `left_join` can be performed to append the numeric scores to the shared document terms. Here, the `left_join`'s `by` parameter needs to declare two different column names as being the shared intersection. The `lastYrTidy` object has a column `term` while the `afinn` object has tokens under the column name `word`. A left join will retain all rows in the left hand table. When words are identified as being shared between the new tables, the AFINN score is appended. When rows of the `lastYrTidy` object are not identified within `afinn`, the rows are retained but columns are filled with `NA`. Table 6.7 is a portion of the `left_join` result to illustrate the filling of NA values.

The NAs within the data can be declared as neutral by first identifying `NA` with `is.na` and then declaring these values as 0. This applies only to the fourth column. The following code nests `is.na` inside of square brackets to the left of the comma so that it checks all rows. To the right of the comma, the integer `4` refers to the `value` column by index position. All of this is to the left of the assignment operator while the replacing value `0` is to the right.

```
afinnJoin[is.na(afinnJoin$value),4] <- 0
```

A `data.frame` can be constructed declaring the `doc` column and another called `polarity`. The `polarity` column is equal to the joined `count` times the `value` columns. Certain posts have more than one count for emotionally scored words. This simply captures not just the occurrence but also the frequency within a document. This

Table 6.7 A selection of the left join table with the polarity values for identified terms.

Document	Term	Count	Value
6	finally	1	NA
6	f*ck	1	−4
6	gave	1	NA
6	injury	1	-2
6	long	1	NA
6	major	1	NA

---

2 Nielsen F. Å. A new ANEW: Evaluation of a word list for sentiment analysis in microblogs. *Proceedings of the ESWC2011 Workshop on 'Making Sense of Microposts': Big things come in small packages 718 in CEUR Workshop Proceedings*, 93–98. 2011 May. http://arxiv.org/abs/1103.2903.

data needs to be aggregated from the individual term level, of which there are more than 26,000 to the document level using `aggregate`. The second code line applies `sum` to `afinnJoinDF` such that the `polarity` column is summed by the unique `doc` identifier.

```
afinnJoinDF <- data.frame(doc = as.numeric(afinnJoin$document),
                          polarity = afinnJoin$count *
afinnJoin$value)
afinnJoinDF <- aggregate(polarity~doc, afinnJoinDF, sum)
```

In order to construct the polarity over time, the original dates need to be appended. First, the `commentDF` object will be made more concise in the `commentDateDF` object. For the polarity over time visual, all other columns are not needed. This employs `data.frame` to create a shared column, `doc`, for intersection along with the original comment date column called `comm_date`. However, the emotional data has been subset to the most recent year using the `idx` object previously. This object is also used here for the same purpose within single square brackets when constructing the concise data frame. The result is a two-column data frame where column one is an identifier and column two is the date it appeared on the forum. The use of `idx` ensures consistency with the text being analyzed.

```
commentDateDF <- data.frame(doc = seq_along(commentDF$id[idx]),
                            comm_date = commentDF$comm_
date[idx])
```

The goal of the additional information is to append the date meta-data to the polarity data frame. This is done with another `left_join` along with the declared shared column `doc`. The result demonstrated in the abridged Table 6.8. Notice how the comments can be spread of multiple days, and with varying polarity. For example, October 2nd, 2020, has a comment labeled as document 1 and a corresponding 0. Subsequently, another comment occurred on October second but with a −1 polarity. Still the sixth document also on October second used more polarizing words resulting in a −10 value. This could have been two uses of a −5 term or any mixture of term and count scores multiplying to −10. To understand the polarity over time another `aggregate` function is applied. Aggregating `polarity` by the `comm_date` column and summing the values with `sum` is executed on the second code line.

```
commentDateDF <- left_join(commentDateDF,
                           afinnJoinDF, by = c('doc'='doc'))
commentDateDF <- aggregate(polarity~comm_date, commentDateDF,
sum)
```

Let's create a new column representing the changing polarity over time. To create the new `cumulativePolarity` function, apply `cumsum` to the original `polarity` column of the aggregated data. This will calculate a running total by date.

```
commentDateDF$cumulativePolarity <- cumsum(commentDateDF$pola
rity)
```

Reviewing the `summary` function call above shows the forum is overtly positive. Although negative language is used, on any given day the totality of language skews toward positive. In fact, only a single day, October 21st had a negative value among the total number of comments for the day, which can be obtained with `which.min` applied to the `polarity` column. This may have been a low commenting day or comments may have used neutral language.

```
summary(commentDateDF)
commentDateDF[which.min(commentDateDF$polarity),]
```

One way to view this data is as a timeline. One could create a rolling average or plot the raw polarity scores on a *y*-axis. This `ggplot` code accepts the polarity data frame and defines the *x*-axis as `comm_date` and `polarity` for the *y*-axis. An empty `geom_line` layer is added to draw the lines followed by a string within `ggtitle` and the predefined High Charts color palettes.

```
ggplot(commentDateDF, aes(x = comm_date, y = polarity)) +
  geom_line() +
  ggtitle('Raw Polarity over time') +
  theme_hc()
```

Another and perhaps more compelling visual would employ the cumulative sum. This lets the audience understand the general positivity of the forum and in reviewing the slope of the cumulative area the velocity of authorship utilizing polarized words. If the slope decreases, either the number of comments decreased, the length of posts shortened, or the words used were more neutral. The overall positive velocity demonstrated in the area chart, Figure 6.6, may signal online community engagement (total area, distance between points) and health (positive slope). As an interactive plot it is easier to realize when there are no posts between dates because the tooltip signal this to the user. Although `echarts4r` can construct a line chart similar to the previous `ggplot` code, the next code chunk purposefully switches to an area chart to add another perspective. Both packages can construct either the line chart or area plot while referring to either `polarity` or `cumulativePolarity`. Notice in Figure 6.6, the following aspects of the forum:

Table 6.8 A selection of comment identifiers, `doc`, the date, and the individual comment's polarity score.

Doc	comm_date	Polarity
1	2020-10-02	0
2	2020-10-03	0
3	2020-10-02	−1
4	2020-10-02	0
5	2020-10-02	0
6	2020-10-02	−10

- There were neutral comments made on 10-21-2020 demonstrated by the slope 0 between 10-11 and 10-12.
- A negative tone was realized on 10-21 because the slope actually decreases from 10-20 to 10-21.
- After a long period of no comments related to "CSK," positive comments reappeared 11-1.
- From day to day the comments add to the positivity as shown with the *overall* upward slope.
- The distance between points can be more than a week so engagement on the "CSK" topic may be diminished. Keep in mind this collection of documents is for a single team. Thus, this forum behavior may be typical or may be different to other teams and search terms.

To construct the visual forward the `commentDateDF` to `e_charts` asserting the *x*-axis as `comm_date`. The `e_area` layer is added indicating that the `cumulative-Polarity` function is the value column. Next, the `gray` theme is applied though any other theme form the package can be utilized. The user slider is added with `e_data-zoom` so a user can zoom into a specific time range. This can be useful for more crowded data, where forum comments occur daily for example. Lastly, the same `e_toolbox_feature` and `e_tooltip` layers are added to give the user more control with the interactive plot.

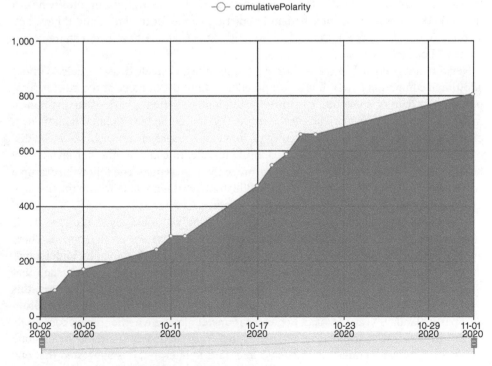

Figure 6.6 The cumulative sum polarity area chart.

```
commentDateDF %>%
  e_charts(comm_date) %>%
  e_area(cumulativePolarity) %>%
  e_theme('gray') %>%
  e_datazoom(type = "slider") %>%
  e_toolbox_feature(feature = "saveAsImage") %>%
  e_tooltip(trigger = 'axis')
```

Another aspect of an online forum is the "social connectivity" of authors by comments. Often authors of posts and comments are not widely spread out among community members. This means many comments occur from a small subset of passionate and engaged forum members. A compelling visual to demonstrate this tendency and identify the most passionate users is called a network graph. Network graphs are set up as nodes and edges. In this use case, a node is a circle, representing a user. The edge is the line connecting the user nodes. Using forum data, a connection is made when two or more users comment on the same thread. More generally, in network graphs, the size of the node may indicate an attribute, the thickness of the edge another attribute, and arrows can even be applied to indicate the direction of the connection for other use cases. As a result, network graphs are used in more than forums; they can be applied to social media with the library `sna` or to other applications like fraud detection where transactions can be identified as groups within the network performed by bad actors. Figure 6.7 shows an example network graph before a more robust one is created with real data. In the figure, user B has commented on threads with users A, C, and D. This user is more central to the overall community health than others. Users A and B have had an interaction on the forum, but E and B have not, so there is no edge between them. Additionally, users C and D have had a shared comment without other users.

Network analysis can be time consuming to compute and create dense visuals. Without additional computing power, it is a best practice to limit the number of records for computation by date or some other feature. Additionally, there are various mathematical methods to lay out a network graph. Conceptually, if each node is a planet with its own gravitational pull based on the number of connecting edges, a network would be displayed so the most active commentor is in the middle. In contrast, another layout may have equal weights for nodes and simply arrange them in a circle. The following example covers network analysis at a cursory level to illustrate what is possible within the realm of sports analytics but it is not an exhaustive example.

After using `subset` on the `commentDF`, where only a single day `2020-11-01` is captured, the `user_network` function from `RedditExtractoR` is applied. There are two parameters which will aid the construction of the network graph and understanding important users in the dialog. First, the `include_author` is a Boolean such that the author is retained within the resulting data object. Depending on the analysis, this may not be useful but here, the goal is to understand the most central figure of the forum on a particular day. Next, the `agg` Boolean parameter dictates whether repeat comments on the same thread are aggregated or kept as additional incremental interactions among users. Since network graphs can be dense and hard to interpret, it is suggested that one first tries `agg = TRUE`.

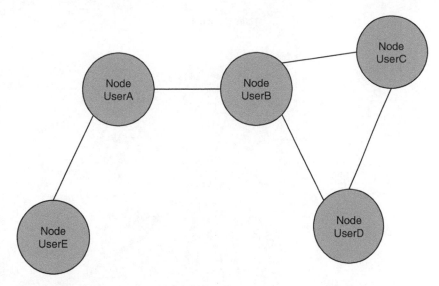

Figure 6.7 An example network graph of user nodes and edge connections.

```
novFirst <- subset(commentDF,
                    commentDF$comm_date=='2020-11-01')
networkGraph <- user_network(novFirst,
                             include_author = T,
                             agg = T)
```

The `networkGraph` object is a list. It contains "edge" and corresponding "node" data frames. Additionally, there are similar objects used in the `igraph` library which is a popular R package for network visuals. These include an "edge list," "igraph object" specific to that package and a plotting object. Thus, one can simply call the `$plot` list element to quickly view the result of calling `user_nework`. Depending on the number of edges and nodes, the visualization may take time to render. The default view is a directed network graph meaning there are arrows when one node comments on another author's thread. Additionally, nodes themselves are scaled by the number of posts resulting in thicker edges. Finally, it is worth noting the result of the default `$plot` call is a JavaScript interactive visual. Therefore, a user can click on an edge to see the comment or highlight a node by clicking on a user. Figure 6.8 demonstrates the central authors for a single day in the forum but does so in a cluttered and hard-to-interpret manner for the purposes of only defining the most central commentors.

```
networkGraph$plot
```

Another option is to extract and manipulate the list elements to reduce the information making the social network visual less cluttered. Of course, this means some information is lost but the goal is to identify super users not necessarily explore the individual comments. First, extract the individual "node" and "edge" data frame from the returns list, `networkGraph`. This is done using the list names but can be done with double square bracket and numeric indexing.

User Network

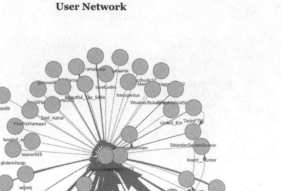

Figure 6.8 The default network plot for a single day's forum interaction.

Table 6.9 A portion of the incident matrix where user "0" commented to user "59," user "0" also commented to user "11" and elsewhere, user "1" commented to user "27."

From	To	Weight	Title	User
0	59	6	"Oh my gawdd Babar and Haider at the crease"	allisonced
0	11	1	"Ugh I know right, this is a mess"	allisonced
...	...	...	...	...
1	27	1	"TBF, it was South Africa in the last..."	babakaalibhed

```
xEdge <- networkGraph$edges
xNode <- networkGraph$nodes
```

Next, create an "incident matrix." This type of matrix demonstrates the interaction between users. The information has not been changed between the two data frames merely structured differently using an `inner_join`. Table 6.9 shows a portion of the join result. Keep in mind the `id` column in `xNode` is numeric but is a unique identifier. Thus, the `from` and `to` columns of the `incidentMatrix` are not values but instead are designations for user screen names in the forum. The table shows an "incident" or interaction between specific users after the `inner_join` is performed declaring the `from` column is keyed to the `id` column between the tables.

```
incidentMatrix <- inner_join(xEdge, xNode, by = c('from'='id'))
```

Next, create a simplified `nodes` data frame with usernames but declare default values and sizes. This helps reduce visual clutter for the audience but does reduce the informative dimensions in the plot. Here, for aesthetics, the values are simply `10` for both the `value` and `size` columns. These can be adjusted to improve aesthetics. R will "recycle" the `10` no matter the length of the `xNode$user` column. Thus, it is not necessary to use `rep` for these data frame vectors.

```
nodes <- data.frame(name = xNode$user,
                    value = 10,
                    size = 10)
```

In addition to nodes, the graph needs a separate "edge" data frame. These vectors can be called directly from the `incidentMatrix` referring to the `from` and `to` columns. Once again many network graphs are "directed" so the default edge data frame needs columns called `source` and `target` though it is not the goal of this analysis.

```
edges <- data.frame(source = incidentMatrix$from,
                    target = incidentMatrix$to)
```

Using `echarts4r` functionality, create a blank `e_charts` layer. This is forwarded to the `e_graph` type. Unlike previous `echarts4r` plots, the data object is not passed into the first layer or type. Instead, each corresponding layer for the nodes and graphs refers to the matching data frames. The blank graph is passed to the `e_graph_nodes` layers referring to the `nodes` data frame. This function is expecting the usernames and the size and values for the circles. Next the `e_graph_edges` layer accepts the `edges` data frame. The `source` and `target` columns refer to the connections between unique users by their identifier, not the author username from the forum. Next, the `e_theme` is declared as `tech-blue` and the user interface for downloading the image is appended. Unlike the previous `echarts4r` plots, there is no need to add a `e_tooltip` layer. By default, the network graph will have username tooltips for mouseovers. Figure 6.9 is a screenshot showing the simplified network graph along with the most central user "CricketMatchBot" as a tooltip.

As the analysis continues to drive down to user level information, it is important to understand not just the users that are prominent in the network graph but the individual positivity or negativity when posting. The following code performs a polarity analysis on the users by performing another `left_join` on the commenting information and the `afinnJoinDF` lexicon. To begin, create `commentDateDF` with `data.frame`. Declare to columns `doc` and `user` with `seq_along` to get a number from one to the length of the `comm_date` vector in `commentDF`. The second column is merely the original `user` column. Then, the `left_join` matches by the document identifier so that each individual document has a scored polarity value.

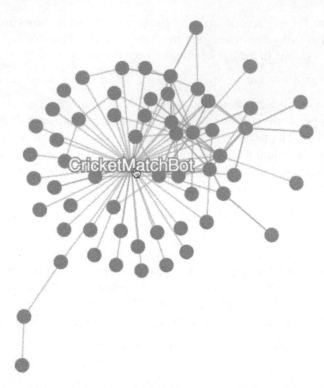

Figure 6.9 The simplified network plot to examine engagement of forum commentors.

```
commentDateDF <- data.frame(doc = seq_along(commentDF$comm_date),
                            user = commentDF$user)
commentDateDF <- left_join(commentDateDF,
                           afinnJoinDF, by = c('doc'='doc'))
commentDateDF <- aggregate(polarity~user, commentDateDF, sum)
```

At this point, the `commentDateDF` object has 11,000 rows among hundreds of unique users. Many of the users have neutral polarity and therefore should be removed from the following examination. To do so, first `aggregate` the data frame. The formula for aggregation is `polarity` by `user` so that the `sum` of polarity is calculated for each user. Although `mean` can be applied instead of `sum`, the following code considers the number of posts along with the polarity scores using temporary data frames. The hope is that the added steps account for short intensely polarized posts balanced against lengthy neutral posts perhaps by the same user. After aggregation, there are still many users, many of which are relatively neutral. The functions `slice_max` and `slice_min` from `dplyr` select `n` rows with the highest or lowest values of a variable. Therefore, the temporary objects `x` and `y` are made to capture the top and bottom 50 users by polarity score. The `%>%` operator forwards the `commentDataDF` object to these functions as is customary in `dplyr`. Next these top and bottom subsets are row bound with `rbind`.

```
x <- commentDateDF %>% slice_max(polarity, n = 50)
y <- commentDateDF %>% slice_min(polarity, n = 50)
z <- rbind(x, y)
```

To account for the number of posts and intensity of the user's forum community contribution, the comment counts by user will be obtained. To begin call `table` on the `user` vector. This is nested in `as.matrix` to change the object type. Next, construct a `data.frame` with a `user` column and `commentCount` from the previous matrix and tally results. Finally, the `rownames` from the `table` call persist as attributes for the final data frame. However, this information is duplicative and is removed in the last code line.

```
commentCount <- as.matrix(table(commentDF$user))
commentCount <- data.frame(user = rownames(commentCount),
                           commentCount= commentCount[,1])
rownames(commentCount) <- NULL
```

Although the `commentCount` object encompasses all unique users, this information needs to be subset and joined to the top and bottom 50 users. The temporary `z` object is left joined to the comment counts according to the `user` column. Then, a new vector `polarityPercomment` is the result of dividing the `polarity` vector by the `commentCount` vector.

```
z <- left_join(z, commentCount, by = c('user'='user'))
z$polarityPerComment <- z$polarity / z$commentCount
```

The following two code executions aid the aesthetics by reordering the data and ensuring the `user` column is a factor. First, `order` is applied to the new `polarityPerComment` column with `decreasing = T` on the left of the comma within square brackets. This reorders the values of the overall data frame. Additionally, the `user` column is declared as a `factor` with the specific ordering in which they appear in the newly reordered data frame rather than the original appearance. The finalized `polarityBars` data frame is used to construct the following visuals.

```
polarityBars <- z[order(z$polarityPerComment,decreasing = T),]

polarityBars$user <- factor(polarityBars$user,
                       levels = unique(as.character
(polarityBars$user)))
```

Since the `ggplot` visual does not have tool tips, another data reduction is needed to avoid a bar chart with over 100 columns. The function `quantile` is applied to the `polarityPerComment` vector along with a floating-point number between 0 and 1. The goal is to identify the lowest and highest deciles in the column. Both are evaluated with a `<` and `>`, respectively. The result is a Boolean vector where TRUE appears if the `polarityPerComment` value is smaller than the 10th percentile and similarly if the value is greater than the top 9th percentile. The two deciles are captured in `bottoms` and `tops`. These two vectors are used as a logical condition within `subset`. The objects are separated by the `|` OR operator. Thus, the `polarityBars` object is subset when the `bottoms` object OR the `tops` object are equal to TRUE. This step is not always needed if the number of users is relatively low and the static plot is easily interpretable.

```
bottoms <- polarityBars$polarityPerComment <
  quantile(polarityBars$polarityPerComment, .1)
tops <- polarityBars$polarityPerComment >
  quantile(polarityBars$polarityPerComment, .9)
topBars <- subset(polarityBars, bottoms|tops==T)
```

Create a `ggplot` passing in the `topBars` data with the *x*-axis as the `user` column, the *y*-axis as the `polarityPerComment`, and a color fill with `polarityPerComment`. Next add the `geom_col` layer. This layer will create bar chart heights according to the values within the data rather than `geom_bar` which makes the height of the bar proposition to the number of cases by group. Thus, `geom_col` is correct because this is an individual behavioral value not tied to a specific group needing a proportional perspective. The `polarityPerComment` values are continuous so color filling could be done with a `scale_fill_gradient` layer determining the `low` and `high` color names. Since usernames can be long, the *x*-axis labels are rotated by 90°, along with a vertical adjustment and a small horizontal change within the `theme` layer. Depending on the usernames, and number of columns in the plot, these values can be adjusted, for example, with 45° angle labels or different vertical heights. Lastly, the overall theme is changed to `theme_hc` along with a declared `ggtittle` to emulate the High Charts color and layout. Figure 6.10 shows the individual forum users sorts by their average polarity. The most and least positive authors can be understood quickly with this visual.

```
ggplot(topBars,
       aes(x = user,
           y = polarityPerComment,
           fill = polarityPerComment)) +
  geom_col() +
  scale_fill_gradient(low = "darkred",
                      high = "darkgreen") +
```

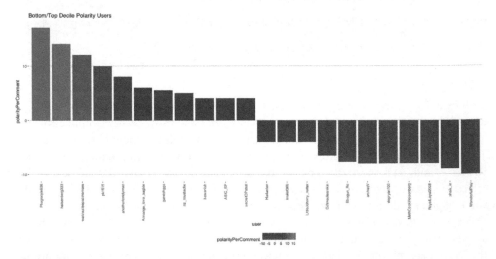

Figure 6.10 The top and bottom decile polarity forum commentors.

```
theme(axis.text.x = element_text(angle = 90,
                                 vjust = 0.5,
                                 hjust=1)) +
theme_hc() + ggtitle('Bottom/Top Decile Polarity Users')
```

Once again, the benefit of a dynamic plot is that a tooltip can help users with untidy data as opposed to removing data. The following code inherits the complete `polarity-Bars` data frame to create an `e_chart` where the *x*-axis is the `user` column. This is passed to the `e_bar` layer declaring `polarityPerComment` as value corresponding to the bar height. Next, the `e_tooltip`, `e_theme`, and `e_toolbox_feature` are added in an object called `pl`.

```
pl <  polarityBars %>%
  e_charts(user) %>%
  e_bar(polarityPerComment) %>%
  e_tooltip() %>%
  e_theme("gray") %>%
  e_toolbox_feature(feature = "saveAsImage")
```

Calling `pl` now will create a gray-themed bar chart for every user in the data frame with corresponding polarity values. An additional layer is added next called `e_visual_map`. This layer explicitly declares behavior regardless of the specific theme. Thus, `pl` is forwarded to the `e_visual_map` layer so that values above 0 are filled green and below 0 are red. The visual map layer needs a parameter for continuous or discrete application of the colors. In this example, the declaration is `piecewise` so the bars are color individually by their relationship to the next parameters. For education purposes, this is deliberately different than the gradient fill employed with `ggplot` though similar color variations could be done with either package. Once declared as `piecewise`, the groupings according to value need to be determined. First for any "piece," or column, greater than 0, the color is explicitly declared as `green`. The `gt` parameter stands for greater than. Next, another parameter is added where `lte` or "less than or equal to" is declared to be color `red`. The tricky part in this layer is knowing the `pieces` input is a list, and that each element of that list is in turn another list with elements as individual values. New programmers to `echarts4r` can easily misplace the closing parentheses or believe only a single list is needed. Figure 6.11 is the result of the `echarts4r` code with declared piecewise coloring.

```
pl %>%
  e_visual_map(
    type = "piecewise",
    pieces = list(
      list(
        gt = 0,
        color = "green"),
      list(
        lte = 0,
        color = "red")))
```

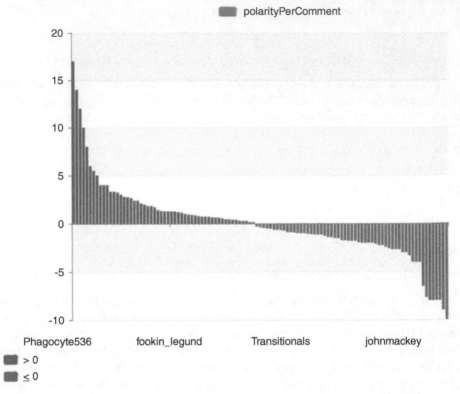

Figure 6.11 The polarity bars with all users. As a user's mouse rolls over a bar, the tooltip shows the specific username and polarity.

Extending the Approaches Employed

There are multiple ways to extend the lessons of this chapter. For example, NLP can employ unsupervised approaches like latent Dirichlet allocation (LDA) topic modeling or deep neural networks in text2vector approaches. These help the practitioner examine topics, themes, and contextual relationships in the corpus. Even more simply you can adjust stop words, sentiment, and polarity lexicons based on your judgment and expertise. These basic adjustments will affect your extracted features and the resulting plots. For example, removing terms like "middle" and "order" will mean the bigram will not be included in the bi-gram word cloud.

Another major way to easily adjust this chapter's lesson is to search for another team in the cricket subreddit. Or if you want to perform these tasks on another sport, or team, simply find the subreddit, or a csv of text using another service like the `twitteR` package enables. The code and its concepts should be easy to apply in new contexts and social media channels like Twitter because the natural language approaches are not specific to cricket or the CSK alone.

In the end, this chapter provides multiple ways to extract insights from fan forums. At one level, the main topics, emotions, and polarity are examined. Then drilling down, the subsequent visuals help identify the drivers of the dialog and the most and least positive and negative users. This chapter is a good starting point though NLP, sentiment, and polarity analysis and even network graphs can be large robust topics individually. Thus, once the general concepts are understood, it is recommended to add fluency by exploring these topics more in depth.

Exercises

1) Describe a social media listening tool. What types of attributes may be insightful?

2) Define polarity.

3) Describe a sentiment lexicon, and that it is useful for.

4) Describe a DTM? What do rows represent? What does it mean to be sparse?

5) Use `get_reddit` with a search term "KKR" for Kolkata Knight Riders.

6) Using the new "KKR" data, create a unigram word cloud in the shape of a circle.

7) Measure the polarity of the overall conversation within the KKR data for the last year.

8) Identify the emotional category with the most identified words among all comments.

9) Identify the most negative KKR commentor among all users.

10) Identify the top positive KKR commentor among all users.

7

Gambling Optimization

Objectives

- Understand the basic premise of sports line ups
- Contextualize the impact of fantasy sports and gambling
- Learn to set a football lineup
- Define a simulation of outcomes
- Solve a linear programming football lineup problem
- Identify a single lineup which maximizes a week's lineup using player point predictions

R Libraries

```
devtools
ffanalytics
rvest
data.table
ggplot2
ggthemes
lpSolve
rPref
echarts4r
rbokeh
```

Similar to Chapter 3, this chapter utilizes an unofficial (at the time of writing) package called `ffanalytics`. The `install_github` function from the `remotes` package is also ported to the `devtools` package. In the code below, the `devtools` function namespace is explicitly called using the double colons. While there is no difference, the use of explicit namespace calls can be useful when functions conflict by name between packages. As a result, namespace calling is demonstrated below to install the GitHub repository package `ffanalytics`.

```
devtools::install_github(repo = "FantasyFootballAnalytics/ffa-
nalytics", build_vignettes = TRUE)
```

Sports Analytics in Practice with R, First Edition. Ted Kwartler.
© 2022 John Wiley & Sons Ltd. Published 2022 by John Wiley & Sons Ltd.

R Functions

```
<-
scrape_data
source
subset
paste
paste0
%>%
html_nodes
html_text
strsplit
unlist
rbind
lapply
rbindlist
make.names
head
inner_join
anti_join
%in%
as.data.frame
as.numeric
median
which
grep
set.seed
ggplot
aes
geom_density
theme_hc
ggtitle
list
for
t
rnorm
data.frame
print
model.matrix
rep
nrow
c
lp
table
```

```
max.col
group_by
count
geom_col
theme
element_text
rownames
order
e_charts
e_bar
e_tooltip
e_toolbox_feature
e_x_axis
e_theme
top_n
facet_grid
facet_wrap
ly_points
filter
psel
low
high
```

Chapter Caveat

This chapter demonstrates a method to analytically select an optimal lineup for a fantasy football team. To begin it must be said that the chapter in no ways promotes gambling nor does it endorse the Draft Kings or similar application. Analytically, lineup selection is an interesting and challenging use case worthy of examination. If you intend to use this chapter's example as a means for gambling, it is provided without endorsement or warranty either implied or explicit.

> If you or someone in your social network suffer from a gambling addiction, the US National Problem Gambling Helpline is 1-800-522-4700. Further, the organization Gambler Anonymous is an international organization that helps individuals recover from gambling problems.

Sports Context

Online fantasy leagues have persisted for more than 20 years in some form or another. In a fantasy sports league, players act as their own general managers forming a fictitious team made of individual athletes. Competitors select athletes in a specific sport to construct a hypothetical team. When the actual athletes play, points are awarded for good performance. Depending on the site and league rules, point assignments vary for athlete actions. A fantasy player's team roster performance is the sum of the individual athlete's actual performance. The difference between reality and fantasy teams is that a fantasy team can be constructed among players across a league not only a single team. For example, a fantasy player may select Baker Mayfield the current Cleveland football team quarter back. When Mayfield throws a pass resulting in a touchdown, 4 points will be awarded to the player's team. Later in the game, Mayfield may throw an interception resulting in a loss of a point. If Mayfield's game ends, the total contribution for the fantasy team is 3 points. Additionally, the fantasy player's roster may include Ezekiel Elliot, the Dallas team's marquee Running Back. When Elliot plays, he may run for 10 yards, which would result in a single point. If that is the extent of his contribution, the player's total fantasy team would include Mayfield's 3 points and Elliot's single point.

Keep in mind, fantasy leagues are not constrained to professional football as shown in this chapter and league administration may be undertaken at multiple sites not just Draft Kings.

Each fantasy league and type of game have corresponding constraints when constructing a roster. For each position points are awarded for different statistics in a game. Overall, this chapter's example demonstrates a typical lineups ruleset. Specifically, a nine-player team must have:

- One quarterback
- Two running backs
- Three wide receivers
- One tight end
- One "Flex" player which could be a running back, wide receiver, or tight end
- One "DST" which is a defensive and special teams' position where points are earned as a unit instead of individually

However, individual athletes have an associated salary cost which fluctuates week to week depending on injuries, opponents, and even weather. The salary cost is dictated by the league administrator. In this chapter's example, a site called Draft Kings. For example, Baker Mayfield may cost $6100 versus a competing quarterback Cam Newton who may be expected to get fewer points but only cost $5400. Thus, an additional constraint to a fantasy player is

- The total salary cost for the roster must be less than or equal to $50,000.

The code in this chapter solves for a particular sport within a particular type of fantasy game. Some games have a different roster makeup, different scoring methodology, or have player assigned in a draft instead of a salary. Care is needed to ensure the code is applicable to a different point schema, roster requirements, and player selection.

Technical Context

In the following code, upcoming week projections are obtained from various online sources. Online sites create point projections in an effort to help fantasy league players but utilize their own models resulting in differences. These projections are assembled and the standard deviation for each is calculated. For example, consider two sites forecasting the upcoming week's points for Baker Mayfield, according to a particular league point schema to be 16.33 and 22.6. Once assembled, the standard deviation of these projections is calculated. A simple example is shown below.

```
sd_pts <- sd(c(16.33, 22.6))
```

In addition, either a weighted or mean average is calculated.

```
avg <- mean(c(16.33, 22.6))
```

Given this information, a simulation can be constructed to emulate the range of possibilities for Baker Mayfield's weekly performance. This assumes a normal distribution with the mean and standard deviations as inputs. Here, 10 games are simulated according to this assumed outcome distribution.

```
tenGames <- rnorm(4, avg, sd_pts)
```

This process can include more than two sites and is applied to hundreds of players. Further, the `rnorm` function in the actual code will simulate 10,000 observations not 4. After significant data manipulation, the results of 10,000 simulated game outcomes among hundreds of players are utilized for linear optimization using the `lpSolve` library.

These inputs are used along with a series of constraints to identify an optimal solution. This process is called linear programming or linear optimization because the constraints have a linear relationship. For example, one constraint is that the roster may only contain nine total players. Thus, a roster's constraint relationship in pseudo code would be `roster player count equals 9`. Similarly, the total roster salary needs to be `less than or equal to 50000`. Consider the following small data frame conceivably from the simulated game point outcomes from `rnorm`.

```
fakeWeekLeague <- data.frame(simGame1 = c(2,7,8,2),
                             simGame2 = c(7,7.5,3,2),
                             simGame3 = c(7,2,8,10),
                             simGame4 = c(1,9,8,2))
rownames(fakeWeekLeague) <- paste0('QBplayer', LETTERS[1:4])
```

A linear optimization could identify the single best player from the data frame from each column. With a single constraint and a small data set, it is easy to identify the best player in `simGame1` is `QBplayerC`, `QBplayerCB` in `simGame2`, and so on. This is because within the respective column outcomes these players are the highest projected points. Of course, there are more constraints than just one and many thousands of columns, but for simplicity, let's assume this data represents only the QB position and that one single player needs to be selected so the constraint is that the `QB roster spot equals one`.

To programmatically identify the optimal player in each of the simulated games of `fakeWeekLeague`, let's select a single same for examination in the object `rosterPossibilities`. This represents the four players' simulated points to choose from.

```
rosterPossibilities <- fakeWeekLeague$simGame4
```

Next, each player counts as a single selection so their cost toward the constraint is one. The liner programming `lp` function requires a matrix so here a matrix of a single row is created. Each player's value toward the selection constraint is one so `1` is repeated four times, one per player. The `playerCost` matrix is the "constraint matrix" used in the upcoming optimization.

```
playerCost <- matrix(c(1, 1, 1,1), nrow=1, byrow=TRUE)
```

At this point, the player possibilities are known as `1,9,8,2` in `simGame4`, represented in `rosterPossibilities`. The cost constraint for each of the four players is one. The direction of the constraint is that the selected value must equal one. This is because only one QB can be selected. For other positions, more spots are accepted so the constraint direction could be less than or equal two or three. With one constraint, the selection is `=` and declared in `direction` below.

```
direction <- c("=")
```

Lastly, the right-hand side of the constraint needs to be declared. With only one spot, it's straight forward that the right-hand side is merely captured in a vector with length one as `1`. One could say the maximum cost to the player selection must be equal to one since the roster needs exactly one QB.

```
maxCost <- c(1)
```

Finally, `lp` is applied to optimize this set of game point possibilities. Here, `lp` is trying to maximize the point potential. Some optimization problems will minimize a cost function. Here, the first input is a string `max`. Next, the vector of possibilities, cost, direction, and right-hand side are passed in. The last parameter is a binary declaration. This is use case specific but since one cannot select a portion of a player and the act of selection is a binary event, this parameter is needed.

```
linearOptimal <- lp("max",
                    rosterPossibilities,
                    playerCost,
                    direction,
                    maxCost,
                    all.bin = TRUE)
```

Once the linear optimization has been run, the solution is obtained by referring to the `solution` element of the object. It is an index of the optimal outcome. Clearly in a vector of `1,9,8,2`, the second player is the correct choice. The code below uses `which` to index the player `rownames` to correctly identify `QBplayerB` as the optimal choice. One can rerun this entire code section referring to another game column by adjusting the `roster-Possibilities` vector.

```
rownames(fakeWeekLeague)[which(linearOptimal$solution==1)]
```

Let's add another constraint to the example. Now let's add player salary costs as another row to the constraint matrix. Now players count toward the QB roster spot as `1` and have a corresponding salary cost. The `playerCost` matrix now has a second for the additional constraint.

```
playerCost <- matrix(c(1, 1, 1,1, 3000,5500,5000,3500), nrow=2,
byrow=TRUE)
```

Now the `direction` object must contain another operator to match the additional row of the `playerCost`. The salary will be less than or equal to a yet-to-be-determined amount on the right-hand side. This linear relationship is demonstrated in the `<=` below within the update vector.

```
direction <- c("=", "<=")
```

Finally, let's assume a fantasy player does not want to spend more than $5000 on the QB position. Thus, not only does any selection count as the roster spot but also the maximum salary amount must be 5000 or less. This is defined in an updated `maxCost` vector to represent values on the right-hand side of the direction operators.

```
maxCost <- c(1, 5000)
```

Applying the same `lp` function will now result in a different player selection for `simGame4`. This is because of the additional constraint.

```
linearOptimal <- lp("max",
                    rosterPossibilities,
                    playerCost,
                    direction,
                    maxCost,
                    all.bin = TRUE)
```

With a single constraint `QBplayerB` was the optimal choice because he had projected nine points. However, the salary cost for this player was 5500. With this additional constraint, player B is dropped because his salary does not satisfy the second constraint where salary is less than or equal to 5000. However, `QBplayerC` satisfies both constraints, where the cost to select is one and the salary is less than or equal to 5000. This is the optimal player because the point value is highest among any remaining players that meet the constraint criteria. The new player is identified as the optimal solution in the code below.

```
rownames(fakeWeekLeague)[which(linearOptimal$solution==1)]
```

The proceeding code applies this concept to hundreds of player, for 10,000 game projections along with 7 constraints. The code concepts are the same as demonstrated in this chapter's selection but care has been taken to illustrate the various data manipulation methods applied to the actual solution.

Complete Code—Linear Programming

To make the code more easily changed week to week, set up basic inputs `wk` and `yr` representing week and year, respectively.

```
wk <- 16
yr <- 2020
```

This code uses the unofficial package `ffanalytics` to obtain data from various fantasy football online sources. This is merely a convenience function, and one could either use `rvest` to scrape data themselves or manually create a CSV file to serve the same purpose. When called, the function will navigate a headless browser to a number of sites such as the URLs below. It is worthwhile to load these or similar manually to understand the data prior to pulling into R. Here `sources` is a vector of string parameters. Considering the package is unofficial, one can use these URLs to build a separate scraping function or manually create files. If this is undertaken, at the very least, these URLs serve as a reference.

- https://www.fantasypros.com/nfl/projections/wr.php
- https://www.fantasysharks.com/apps/bert/forecasts/projections.php?League=-1&scoring=1&uid=4&Segment=707&Position=6
- https://www.cbssports.com/fantasy/football/stats/QB/2020/16/projections/nonppr
- https://www.numberfire.com/nfl/fantasy/fantasy-football-projections/rb
- https://www.fleaflicker.com/nfl/leaders?statType=7&sortMode=1&position=8&tableOffset=0

This code will obtain values from two sites but has additional sites commented out for reference. Additionally, care must be taken because the `scrape_data` function is an abstraction meaning it could inadvertently obtain the wrong statistics like seasonal data will have a cascading effect on the rest of the code. This chapter's example uses just two sources which have been verified while the others have different pointing schema resulting in inflated player point projections. Lastly, using only two sources greatly simplifies the code to aid learning.

```
sources <- c('FantasySharks', 'NumberFire') #'Yahoo' 'Fantasy-
Data' 'CBS' 'FantasyPros' 'FleaFlicker'
```

Once the `sources` are created, the object is passed as the first parameter to `scrape_data`. Since the goal is a complete lineup, the `pos` parameter defaults to all player positions in a fantasy football lineup. The last two parameters refer to the top level `wk` and `yr` inputs.

```
scrape <- scrape_data(src = sources,
                      pos = c('QB', 'RB', 'WR', 'TE', 'DST', 'K'),
                      season = yr,
                      week = wk)
```

Each of the many online fantasy football leagues has varying point schema. In this example, the current Draft Kings website points are declared in a named list. Other popular sites like Fan Duel and Yahoo may have different point structures so care must be taken to ensure this is correct. At the time of writing, the Draft King daily fantasy football scoring can be obtained at https://www.draftkings.com/help/rules/nfl. The code below creates `DKscoring` with elements `pass`, `rush`, `rec` (receiving), `misc` (miscellaneous), `ret` (returns), `kick`, `dst` (defense and special teams), and finally a `pts_bracket` defining thresholds for points allowed for defense and special teams. This object can be overwhelming if not taken little by little. The package author provides a guide for scoring settings which can be called upon in console with `vignette("scoring_settings")`. According to the vignette, the code of this object is optional because there is a default scoring parameter if a customized list is not provided later in the code.

```
DKscoring <- list(
  pass = list(
    pass_att = 0, pass_comp = 0, pass_inc = 0,
    pass_yds = 0.04, pass_tds = 4, pass_int = -1,
    pass_40_yds = 0, pass_300_yds = 3, pass_350_yds = 0,
    pass_400_yds = 0),
  rush = list(
    all_pos = TRUE, rush_yds = 0.1, rush_att = 0,
    rush_40_yds = 0, rush_tds = 6, rush_100_yds = 3,
    rush_150_yds = 0, rush_200_yds = 0),
  rec = list(
    all_pos = TRUE,
    rec = 1, rec_yds = 0.1, rec_tds = 6,
    rec_40_yds = 0, rec_100_yds = 3, rec_150_yds = 0,
    rec_200_yds = 0),
  misc = list(
    all_pos = TRUE, fumbles_lost = -1, fumbles_total = 0,
    sacks = 0, two_pts = 2),
  ret = list(
    all_pos = TRUE, return_tds = 6, return_yds = 0),
  kick = list(
    xp = 1.0, fg_0019 = 3.0, fg_2029 = 3.0,
    fg_3039 = 3.0, fg_4049 = 4.0, fg_50 = 5.0,
    fg_miss = 0.0),
  dst = list(
    dst_fum_rec = 2, dst_int = 2, dst_safety = 2,
    dst_sacks = 1, dst_td = 6, dst_blk = 2,
    dst_ret_yds = 0, dst_pts_allowed = 0),
  pts_bracket = list(
    list(threshold = 0, points = 10),
    list(threshold = 1, points = 7),
    list(threshold = 7, points = 4),
    list(threshold = 14, points = 1),
    list(threshold = 21, points = 0),
    list(threshold = 28, points = -1),
    list(threshold = 35, points = -4)))
```

A best practice to improve code auditing and conciseness is to save the above scoring schema as a separate R file. This abstracts away the complex list code so it can be called with the base-R function `source`. As long as pointing does not change often, then this is an acceptable method to reduce the number of lines in a script. Below is an example where the above Draft King score list has been saved as a file `dkScoring.R`. It is then called with `source` and the explicit path. This reduces ~40 lines of code to one. Considering the point schema is unlikely to change week to week and that one may want to have multiple scoring files for each site, this is a suggested practice.

```
source('~/Desktop/SportsAnalytics/manuscripts/c7/dkScoring.R')
```

Table 7.1   A portion of the player point projection table demonstrating three average types.

Id	First name	Last name	Team	Position	Average type	Points	Sd. pts.
13590	Baker	Mayfield	CLE	QB	Weighted	18.32	1.75
13591	Josh	Rosen	SFO	QB	Average	1.68	NA
13592	Sam	Darnold	CAR	QB	Robust	15.28	1.40

Once the data has been obtained with `scrape_data` and the scoring rules defined in a list, one can obtain player projections with `projections_table`. Once projections are made another function, `add_player_info` appends the first and last names along with team. Otherwise, the projections table only has a unique `id` column. Among other variables, each player is assigned three types of point averages based on the spread of projections from the online web scrape and a standard deviation from the online projections. The function returns a column `avg_type` declaring each average type. Table 7.1 is a portion of the `proj` table with added player information.

```
proj <- projections_table(scrape, scoring_rules = DKscoring)
proj <- add_player_info(proj)
```

> Keep in mind this analysis accepts these projection and standard deviations directly. This assumes the website projections are sound. One could possibly improve the results by employing their own point projection model. For example, a machine learning model could provide both point estimates and confidence intervals for a player's projected points that may be more accurate than what is prescribed here. However, this chapter is fundamentally about the mechanics of a linear programming solution, so the default behavior is accepted. Throughout the code, the projected values column, 'points', is called out should a reader want to deviate from the default projects within this table.

The next step is to obtain a single average type for use in the analysis. Thus, the `subset` function is applied to the `avg_type` column referring to `robust`. Next, an additional player full name column is appended called `player` on the left of the assignment operator. On the right-hand side, the `paste` function concatenates the `first_name` column with the `last_name` separated by a single space. This column is useful later when joining data rather than manually matching.

```
avg         <- subset(proj, proj$avg_type=='robust')
avg$player <- paste(avg$first_name, avg$last_name, sep = ' ')
```

Next, the week's salaries need to be obtained. Some online practitioners of the linear optimization lineup method advocate for exporting this data from the Draft Kings lineup page manually.[1] However, using `rvest`'s `read_html` function, it is possible to programmatically collect salary information. One such site called www.rotoguru1.com is utilized below.

---

1 Miles, A. (2019, September 20). *Building Optimal Daily Fantasy Lineups in R.* Aaron's Analytics Blog.https://amiles.netlify.app/2019/09/building-optimal-daily-fantasy-lineups-in-r.

To begin, create a string variable by concatenating without spaces utilizing the `paste0` command. The parameters of the URL construction include the top-level variables `yr` and `wk`. Once constructed the URL can be tested by copying and pasting the complete URL into a web browser. At the time of publication this website URL, if properly formatted, will load a table where data is semicolon delimited. Of course, this is just a single example webpage, another site with salary data could be web scraped or as Aaron Miles[2] suggested in his blog manually recorded to ensure accuracy and consistency.

```
salariesURL <- paste0('http://rotoguru1.com/cgi-bin/fyday.
pl?week=',wk,
                        '&year=', yr,
                        '&game=dk&scsv=1')
salariesURL
```

Next, use the `read_html` function so R will create a headless browser and download the HTML. The `rvest` library is from the tidy-verse so the next code line follows that coding style to apply `html_nodes` and `html_text` in succession. The `html_nodes` function determines what area of the HTML document should be selected using the "x-path" language. Next, the text is then selected from that node with `html_node` as opposed to an HTML attribute.

```
salaries <- read_html(salariesURL)
salaries <- salaries %>% html_nodes(xpath = '//pre') %>% html_
text()
```

As with many web scraping efforts, the result is messy and needs to be manipulated to become useful. The line return character byte string is often encoded as `/n` when parsed by R. At this point, the salaries data is a large single character string with line returns embedded. Thus, applying `strsplit` will string split the single character object whenever the pattern `/n` is matched. The result is a list because a `strsplit` may yield a ragged, uneven object. However, in this case, each line of the data frame is complete and there is a single-line return at the end. Hence, simply applying the `unlist` function will create the rows of the data. Now that the object is a string vector instead of a single running character string, the `strsplit` function is employed again to break up each individual element of the vector. This time the pattern is a semicolon `;` instead of the more typical comma. Unfortunately, this string split converts the object back to a list, so the string manipulation is not quite ready.

```
salaries <- strsplit(salaries, '\n')
salaries <- unlist(salaries)
salaries <- strsplit(salaries, ';')
```

To understand how the data has been manipulated, let's review a single record of the resulting salaries. If one calls the 33rd element of the list through indexing, the object type is a string vector with length 10. The vector can be organized into a matrix by simply

---

2 Miles, A. (2019, September 20). *Building Optimal Daily Fantasy Lineups in R.* Aaron's Analytics Blog.https://amiles.netlify.app/2019/09/building-optimal-daily-fantasy-lineups-in-r.

Table 7.2 A single player's salary information from the web scrape.

[,1]	[,2]	[,3]	[,4]	[,5]	[,6]	[,7]	[,8]	[,9]	[,10]
"16"	"2020"	"1528"	"Mayfield, Baker"	"QB"	"cle"	"a"	"nyj"	"10"	"6100"

calling `rbind` on this single list element. The result is shown in Table 7.2. Keep in mind that all elements are technically character strings even if they appear to be numeric or categorical.

```
salaries[[33]]
rbind(salaries[[33]])
```

So, the first step to organize the `salaries` object is by employing `lapply`. This lets a function be applied to each element of a list and returns a list of the same length. Here, `rbind` is applied so each list element mimics Table 7.2. Next, another `lapply` all is applied so that each list element is converted to a `data.frame`. At this point there is a list where each individual element is a one row data frame.

```
salaries <- lapply(salaries, rbind)
salaries <- lapply(salaries, data.frame)
```

The problematic issue is that the string vector lengths differ from list element to list element. This can occur if the data is incomplete or when a different player position does not have all appropriate information, for example, if a data frame is web scraped that has an age column, but the age variable is not applicable to an entire defensive or special team unit. As a list of data frames, the `data.table` function `rbindlist` can be used to flatten the objects to a single data frame. This is similar to `do.call(rbind, some_list)` but has two noticeable differences. First, the function is optimized to be much fast than a base-R implementation. Second, the additional parameter `fill = TRUE` will fill in column values with NA. This solves the issue described earlier where the number of columns may not be consistent.

```
salaries <- rbindlist(salaries, fill = T)
```

It turns out for this particular web page the first row of the flattened data frame contains the column names. To capture this information, the `names` need to be declared on the left of the assignment operator. On the right side, the `make.names` function is applied to the first row declared with a squared bracket index to the left of the comma. The `make.names` function cleans the strings syntactically. If a column name has a space such as "DK points," it is made to be syntactically valid as "DK.points" with `make.names`. The second code line simply drops the first row since it does not contain player information and is no longer needed since the values were declared as column names instead. The result of this entire effort is a consistent data frame object which can be examined with by calling a few rows as shown in the third line of code. This has been captured in Table 7.3. Since the first row was removed, the player Baker Mayfield's index position has moved up.

Table 7.3 A portion of the cleaned up player salary data after being web scraped.

Week	Year	GID	Name	Pos	Team	h.a	Oppt	DK.Points	DK.salary
16	2020	1528	Mayfield, Baker	QB	cle	a	nyj	10	6100
16	2020	1378	Newton, Cam	QB	nwe	h	buf	9.76	5400
16	2020	1551	Tagovailoa, Tua	QB	mia	a	lvr	8.86	5400

```
names(salaries) <- make.names(salaries[1,])
salaries        <- salaries[-1,]
salaries[32:34,]
```

The upcoming code seeks to perform an inner join between projected player statistics and the cost in Draft Kings salary for the player. An inner join acts to append columns when rows are shared by a unique identifier. For example, consider a table that has a row with ID "playerA" along with a corresponding "height" column. Another table has two rows, "playerA" and "playerB." This second table has a column "weight." If an inner join is performed on the two tables, first the rows in common are identified by the ID, specifically "playerA." Then *both* columns are retained so that the playerA's attributes for height and weight are returned.

As shown in the `Name` column of `salaries`, the structure is "last name comma first name." This column needs to be separated into first and last names so that a match can be obtained with the player projections. Although one could manually match player projections to the scraped salaries, the code below will perform an `inner_join`. The tradeoff is that a join only matches when the values are exactly the same while a manual review could ensure all players are accounted for. At its core, this is a speed versus accuracy tradeoff often seen when coding and data manipulation in particular. This is up to the practitioner and is shown as an example though additional string matching could be done including a "fuzzy match" instead of an `inner_join`.

Using `strsplit` on the `Name` vector with the splitting pattern `,` will separate the last name from the first name in a list. Since it is a list, the `lapply` function is needed to apply `tail` to each element in the second line of code. In this example, the `1` represents the `n` parameter of `tail` so that the last string of each list element is selected. The result is still a list but one where only a single character string has been retained. Thus, simply calling `unlist` on the object will change the class to a simple character vector. These steps could be nested into a single line not requiring a temporary, `tmpFirstName` object but are separated here to aid in learning. The unlisted vector is appended in a new column called `firstName` declared on the left of the assignment operator.

```
tmpFirstName       <- strsplit(salaries$Name, ', ')
tmpFirstName       <- lapply(tmpFirstName, tail, 1)
salaries$firstName <- unlist(tmpFirstName)
```

Similar code is then applied to obtain the player last names. The difference is that the `head` function is called to return the first `n` observations of the `strsplit` list. Here, `n` is still `1` to return only the first value. Although using head to obtain the last name may be confusing, the original `Name` column is "last name comma first name," so the `head` function will obtain the last name as the first element of the split string.

```
tmpLastName         <- strsplit(salaries$Name, ',')
tmpLastName         <- lapply(tmpLastName, head, 1)
salaries$lastName <- unlist(tmpLastName)
```

Next, an `inner_join` is applied to the `avg` player projections as the "left hand table" and the `salaries` web scrape as the "right hand table." However, the `DST` position is unique compared to the other rows. The `DST` position does not have traditional first and last name identifiers, so the join is only performed on the `first_name` to `firstName` key columns. Thus, the first join is performed on a `subset` of the `avg` object where the `position` column equals `DST` and another `subset` of `salaries` when the `Pos` column equals `Def`. The join declares a `defenses` data frame with the projections and salaries only for the defense and special team "position."

```
defenses <- inner_join(subset(avg, avg$position=='DST'),
                       subset(salaries, salaries$Pos =='Def'),
                       by = c('first_name'= 'firstName'))
```

Next, another `inner_join` is performed for the remaining positions. Now the code is changed so the `subset` negates the `DST` position utilizing the `!` operator. The non-DST positions represent the left-hand table. The `salaries` table remains the right-hand table without any need to subset because an inner join will drop non-shared rows. Since players have both first and last names, there are two identification variables. On the left, the `first_name` and `last_name` equate to the `firstName` and `lastName`, respectively. When both conditions are shared explicitly, the join is performed to append the salary information. Both are needed because some first and last names alone may be shared among multiple players for common names like the last name "Brown" which appears nine times.

```
players <- inner_join(avg,
                      salaries,
                      by = c('first_name'= 'firstName',
                             'last_name' = 'lastName'))
```

This join only works if the first and last names are shared explicitly. Name suffixes such as ".Jr" may make the join misidentify a player. Still, in this case nearly 400 of the original players in the projection table were identified. One could review the players that were dropped in an effort to clean up the names or just append the salary information manually. To identify the unmatched players, the `anti_join` function is helpful. The `anti_join` removes rows in the left-hand table if a matching row was identified in the right-hand table. The result is the unmatched players for review.

```
droppedPlayers <- anti_join(avg,
                            salaries,
                            by = c('first_name'= 'firstName',
                                   'last_name' = 'lastName'))
```

This code simply ignores the unmatched athletes because programmatic matching is faster and less error prone. When employing this code with actual monetary implications, fixing the `droppedPlayers` object with salary data is warranted. If performed, simply `rbind` the data to the `allPos` object constructed below.

Since the `defenses` object was not joined on the `last_name = lastName`, the columns do not match between `defenses` and `players`. To rectify this missing column, append a `lastName` column of `NA` to the `players` data frame. R will recycle the `NA` for all rows so there is no need to use a repeating function like `rep`. Alternatively, the `lastName` column could be dropped from the `defenses` object by declaring it as `NULL`. Once the columns are match between the two tables, the `players` and `defenses` data frames are row-bound with `rbind` in the `allPos` object.

```
players$lastName <- NA
allPos <- rbind(players, defenses)
```

The next step is to simulate many games for each player recording the possible point outcomes. Let's perform the operation on a single player before expanding to all players. To do so, select the relevant variables from the `allPos` data. Within square brackets to the right of the comma, use the `%in%` operator with the column names of `allPos` and a vector of strings representing column headers to retain. The lineups data frame now contains the name, position, projected points, actual point results, weekly salary cost, and the standard deviation for the predicted points. This chapter uses predicted outcomes although as a historical lookback the `DK.points` are known. These actual outcomes are retained here for comparison but in a forward-looking analysis would not be available. Next, the object class is changed to `data.frame` with `as.data.frame` to ensure functions behave as expected. Otherwise, the object also has the table "tbl" object class which can cause errors with some functions.

```
lineups <- allPos[,names(allPos) %in%
                  c('Name', 'position', 'points',
                    'DK.points','DK.salary', 'sd_pts')]
lineups <- as.data.frame(lineups)
```

To avoid potential issues where a column can be considered a character string, the following code explicitly declares the `DK.salary`, `DK.points`,`points`, and `sd_pts` columns as numeric. This may not be needed depending on the web page and prior data manipulation but is good practice when the data has been obtained from many webpages and manipulated significantly.

```
lineups$DK.salary <- as.numeric(lineups$DK.salary)
lineups$DK.points <- as.numeric(lineups$DK.points)
lineups$points    <- as.numeric(lineups$points)
lineups$sd_pts    <- as.numeric(lineups$sd_pts)
```

Some of the projection data have `sd_pts` as NA. One could remove these players as incomplete observations using `complete.cases`, set the standard deviation to 0 so that the projected points do not vary in the simulation or the values for these players can be imputed. The code below identifies NA in the `sd_pts` vector with `is.na` on the left of the assignment operator. The `is.na` Boolean response TRUE is replaced with the right side of the assignment operator function. On the right side, the `median` is calculated among all players with the additional parameter of `na.rm = TRUE`. There are multiple methods for imputation such as using a model or using the median by position, but this code suffices as a simplistic approach.

```
lineups$sd_pts[is.na(lineups$sd_pts)]<- median(lineups$sd_pts,
na.rm = T)
```

Additionally, the following code does not run if the `points` and `DK.salary` values are 0. As a result, the next code line drops any rows where this is the case. Using indexing to the left of the comma, the function `which` identifies any rows where one or more logical conditions occur. In this case, the `points` and `DK.salary` columns both must be greater than 0. If both conditions are met the row is retained. Table 7.4 is the result of calling `head` on the `lineups` object after imputation and removal of inconsistent rows.

```
lineups <- lineups[ which(lineups$points > 0 &
                          lineups$DK.salary >0), ]
head(lineups)
```

Now that the data has been made more concise and properly corrected, let's examine a simulation for a single player. First create a single player object `onePlayer`. This is done by using `grep` which is a regular expression pattern match function. The function is searching for the string pattern "Baker" within the `Name` column. The result is the row integer where the pattern is identified. Since this is to the left of the comma, the single row is returned. Next, for consistency in this code, a seed is set for the next function. In practical application, the `set.seed` is not needed.

```
onePlayer <- lineups[grep('Baker', lineups$Name),]
set.seed(1234)
```

Table 7.4 The smaller player data set with projected points, standard deviation of the projections, name, actual outcome points, and weekly salary cost. Some standard deviation values have been imputed resulting in a repeating value.

Position	Points	Sd_pts	Name	DK.points	DK.salary
QB	17.52	1.18	Brees, Drew	13.14	5900
QB	21.00	0.84	Brady, Tom	32.92	6800
TE	2.90	1.18	Witten, Jason	3.2	2500
WR	7.35	1.18	Fitzgerald, Larry	8.80	3400
QB	13.53	1.18	Rivers, Philip	12.80	5600
QB	15.81	0.23	Roethlisberger, Ben	28.48	6400

To simulate 10,000 games from this player, the `rnorm` function is applied. The first parameter is `n` where the number of observations, `10000` is declared. Next, the `mean` parameter is represented as the projected points in the `points` column. Lastly, the player's standard deviation is provided. The result is 10,000 observations representing a normal distribution where the mean is projected points for the player and the standard deviation contributes to the distribution kurtosis. This data is captured in a single column data frame called `singlePlayerPts` because the `rnorm` results are nested in `as.data.frame`. As a data frame the column name is explicitly declared as `ptsDist` with the `names` function on the left side of the assignment operator. The simulated distribution has a range from 12.07 to 24.96 points meaning this player could score as few as 12.07 points but also as many as 24.96, although these extreme values are unlikely.

```
singlePlayerPts <- as.data.frame(rnorm(10000,
                                        onePlayer$points,
                                        onePlayer$sd_pts))
names(singlePlayerPts) <- 'ptsDist'
```

Figure 7.1 is a kernel density plot to understand the distribution of the player's simulated 10,000 games. Using `ggplot` pass in the `rnorm` data frame. The aesthetics are declared as the `ptsDist` variable. The next layer, `geom_density` adds the density distribution. The last

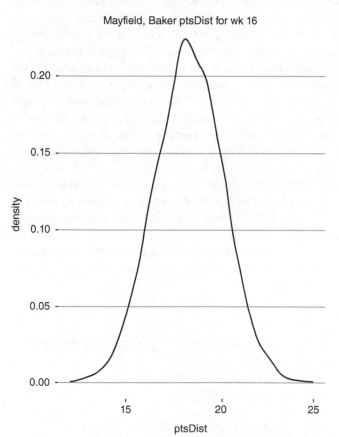

Mayfield, Baker ptsDist for wk 16

Figure 7.1 The "Baker Mayfield" point distribution of 10,000 simulated games where the average is 18.32.

two layers change the overall theme to High Charts and apply a dynamically declared title using `paste` referring to the `Name` column and the `wk` variable.

```
ggplot(singlePlayerPts, aes(x = ptsDist)) +
  geom_density() +
  theme_hc() +
  ggtitle(paste(onePlayer$Name, 'ptsDist for wk', wk))
```

Setting aside the single player's example, the following code will apply the same principle for all players. In the end, all players will have 10,000 simulated games where the average is the projected points, and the standard deviation is individual player's value. To begin, a variable `nGames` declares the number of observations to construct. Next an empty list is instantiated called `gameOutcomes`.

```
nGames        <- 10000
gameOutcomes <- list()
```

The loop begins with the `for` function. This will repeat the code inside the curly brackets a specific number of times. In this case, the variable `i` will iterate from one to the number of rows in `lineups` object. Within the loop the `onePlayer` data frame is recreated with an index value according to the `i` variable. The first time the loop executed `i` equals one, after the loop completes it restarts with `i` equal to two. The `i` variable will iterate until `i` reaches the number of rows in `lineups`. The `rnorm` function is applied as shown previously to simulate 10,000 game outcomes for the specific player. When this code is run the resulting observation draws will differ slightly than the proceeding tables but the overall distribution mean and standard deviation will be consistent. These values are transposed with the `t` function. Now when `as.data.frame` is applied, a single row with 10,000 columns is created as opposed to the previous single player example. The functional operation is the same, but the data has a changed orientation aiding the overall construction for all players. Next the `names` function is used to declare the 10,000 columns. The `paste0` function concatenates the string `game` to a vector of numbers 1 to 10,000 without spaces. Now each column has a unique simulated game identifier. These 10,000 simulated columns are appended in the `simPts` data frame along with the original player data. The `simPts` data frame contains one row with 10,006 columns of player information and simulated game outcomes. It is then added as an element in the `gameOutsomes` list using the `i` element as a double bracketed index `[[i]]`. The last line of the loop is not mandatory but does print a player's name and the `i` value to console. This can help the practitioner know the loop has not frozen the R session and that progress is being made.

```
for(i in 1:nrow(lineups)){
  onePlayer <- lineups[i,]
  simPts <- t(rnorm(nGames, onePlayer$points, onePlayer$sd_pts))
  simPts <- as.data.frame(simPts)
  names(simPts) <- paste0('game', 1:nGames)
  simPts <- data.frame(onePlayer, simPts)
  gameOutcomes[[i]] <- simPts
  print(paste('working on player:',lineups$Name[i], i))
}
```

At this point, the list `gameOutcomes` has a single row data frame for all players. Once again the `rbindlist` function will flatten this object to over 400 rows and 10,006 columns. To understand the new data object, examine Table 7.5 which is called with the second line of code. Keep in mind the first 10 columns are shown but the object contains many thousands.

```
gameOutcomes <- rbindlist(gameOutcomes)
gameOutcomes[190:194,1:10]
```

To find a linear solution, a "constraint" matrix needs to be constructed. This is a dummy variable matrix for the positions. The following code applied to a portion of the data aids in understanding the data manipulation which is applied to the *entire* data set later. It is not actually used in the functional code for the linear programming solutions. The first line calls head with an `n` equal to `5` to review five rows. The `model.matrix` function expands factors to a set of dummy variables. In this case, only the variable `position` is used to create dummy variables using the data shown in Table 7.5. The newly created dummy variable matrix is shown in Table 7.6. Notice Table 7.5 has four QB positions and one RB. This information is captured as a set of dummy variables in Table 7.6. This operation is often referred to as one-hot encoding. There would be more columns for other positions if the original `position` variable in the small selection contained more than two factor levels. When applied broadly there are five columns, one per position.

```
head(model.matrix(~ position + 0,gameOutcomes[190:194,]),5)
```

Table 7.5 A portion of the player data with appended simulated game outcomes.

Position	Points	Sd_pts	Name	DK.points	DK.salary	Game1	Game2	Game3	Game4
QB	23.03	0.92	Allen, Josh	35.30	7300	23.82	22.67	23.87	23.47
QB	18.31	1.83	Mayfield, Baker	10.00	6100	19.37	17.78	18.95	20.80
QB	15.28	1.40	Darnold, Sam	17.00	5000	16.41	13.69	16.69	15.84
QB	22.82	0.64	Jackson, Lamar	22.32	8000	21.60	23.46	23.80	23.45
RB	5.80	3.32	Michel, Sony	6.90	4500	1.80	7.83	5.27	1.20

Table 7.6 The one hot encoding for the position variable from Table 7.5.

positionQB	positionRB
1	0
1	0
1	0
1	0
0	1

Table 7.7 The transposed dummy variable matrix for a small portion of the 'position' variable.

	190	191	192	193	194
positionDST	0	0	0	0	0
positionQB	1	1	1	1	0
positionRB	0	0	0	0	1
positionTE	0	0	0	0	0
psotitionWR	0	0	0	0	0

In the actual solution code, this modeling matrix is transposed in Table 7.7 using the 't' function. As with any transposition, the data values are not changed merely the orientation of the object. Now the rows are represented as numbered columns.

```
t(model.matrix(~ position + 0,gameOutcomes))[,190:194]
```

Now that the basic manipulation is understood, let's construct the larger one-hot encoded matrix. To construct the constraint matrix, use 'rbind' with the transposed 'position' variable similar to the previous example. The second row bound object uses 'rep' to repeat the number '1' for all game outcomes. This will represent the player count for each position. For example, using three WRs will need to be accounted for as 1 + 1 + 1. The last element to be row bound is the player salary information. In total this represents the constraint matrix used later.

```
conMat <- rbind(t(model.matrix(~ position + 0,gameOutcomes)),
                rep(1, nrow(gameOutcomes)),
                gameOutcomes$DK.salary)
```

Some basic attribute information is needed to keep the data easily understood. Since the last two items were appended without row names, the attributes are declared below. The 'rownames' function is used to access the object attributes of a matrix. Here the sixth and seventh values are replaced using the combine, 'c', function with the two denoting strings. Next, the column names are made syntactically correct with 'colnames' on the left side of the assignment operator and 'make.names' on the right hand side. Finally, a familiar part of the object is demonstrated in Table 7.8. Notice the players are the same as before, the position data has been encoded, each player's count is set to one, and each corresponding salary value is captured in the last row. The total constraint matrix has seven rows and more than 400 columns, one per player.

```
rownames(conMat)[6:7] <- c('playerCount', 'salary')
colnames(conMat) <- make.names(gameOutcomes$Name)
conMat[1:7,190:194]
```

The next object in the linear optimization solution accounts for the 10,000 game outcomes among all players. As an illustrative example, let's select a single game out of the 10,000. Here the 'gameOutcomes' object limited to only 'game2022' value. This 'game2022' string is passed on the right side of the comma checking the column 'names' within square brackets. A consequence of the previous 'rbindlist' function is that the object is both a

Table 7.8 The encoded data, showing a player counts as a specific position, is counted against a lineup position limit and has a corresponding salary cost.

	Allen.Josh	Mayfield.Baker	Darnold.Sam	Jackson.Lamar	Michel.Sony
positionDST	0	0	0	0	0
positionQB	1	1	1	1	0
positionRB	0	0	0	0	1
positionTE	0	0	0	0	0
positionWR	0	0	0	0	0
playerCount	1	1	1	1	1
Salary	7300	6100	5000	8000	4500

`data.frame` and `data.table` class. On one hand, this helps make the code computation fast but this also means some typical operations do not work as a base-R object. Here, the third parameter, `with = FALSE` allows the object to only be treated as a data frame. As a result, the base-R indexing works as expected. The result is a one column data frame and data table object representing the player point distributions for the 2022 observation of the `rnorm` distribution run previously.

```
entireLeaguePlay <- gameOutcomes[, (names(gameOutcomes) ==
'game2022'), with=F]
```

Next, the player names are appended to align to the previous demonstration tables. A simple two column data frame is constructed with `data.frame` declaring the `player` column as the `Name` vector and the single 2022 vector from the previous code. This second column is names `simPts`. Table 7.9 shows the familiar players and their simulated point outcomes for a single game. When the complete optimization is run all 10,000 games are examined as individual sets of outcomes where there is one linear optimization for each game 1 to 10,000.

```
exampleSingleWk <- data.frame(player = gameOutcomes$Name,
                              position = gameOutcomes$position,
                              salary = gameOutcomes$DK.salary,
                              simPts = entireLeaguePlay)
exampleSingleWk[190:194,]
```

Table 7.9 Where Baker Mayfield's game points were simulated to be 20.14. This is merely one game scenario among 10,000.

Player	Position	Salary	Game2022
Allen, Josh	QB	7300	23.97
Mayfield, Baker	QB	6100	20.14
Darnold, Sam	QB	5000	16.76
Jackson, Lamar	QB	8000	22.84
Michel, Sony	RB	4500	4.78

Before a single `game2022` solution can be identified, the direction matrix needs to be constructed. Here the data frame `lineupDF` is constructed to organize the input directions. Overall, the data must be in the same order as the constraint matrix row attributes. The `position` column is not really needed but is used to ensure the ordering of the following two column values are as expected. The next column, `lineupNeed`, declares the threshold and the final column `directionConstraints` determines the direction of the threshold to be optimized. Although the code may be less well understood, Table 7.10 shows the object concisely. In the end, the linear programming solution will attempt to find a solution that solves for all inputs according to the declared direction in this table according to the constraints table made previously where the values are supplied as the simulated game points.

```
lineupDF <- data.frame(position = c('positionDST', 'positionQB',
                                    'positionRB', 'positionTE',
                                    'positionWR',
'totalPlayersLineup', 'maxSalary'),
                          lineupNeed = c(1,1,3,2,4,9, 50000),
                          directionConstraints =
c('=','=','<=','<=','<=','=','<='))
```

```
lineupDF
```

In the end, an optimization will be run to *maximize* the points for an individual game. Additional right-hand directions can be added as long as there are corresponding constraints dummy variables in the constraint matrix. This example uses `game2022` whereby the optimization adheres to the following constraints and corresponding directions:

- One Defensive Special Teams Group is selected
- One Quarter Back is selected
- Up to three Running Backs are selected
- One Tight End is selected
- Up to four Wide Receivers are selected
- The total lineup is equal to nine players
- The total salary amount is less than or equal to 50,000

Table 7.10 The lineup attributes along with the direction to be optimized.

Position	lineupNeed	directionConstraints
positionDST	1	=
positionQB	1	=
positionRB	3	≤
positionTE	1	=
positionWR	4	≤
totalPlayersLineup	9	=
maxSalary	50,000	≤

The following code applies the linear optimization function `lp` to a single game outcome. The first input is the type of optimization sought, either minimization or maximization. In this use case, the goal is maximizing the lineup points for a simulated game; hence, `max` is passed as a string. Next, the point values for a single game are accepted. This refers to the single column where all 400 plus players' simulated point totals are captured in `game2022`. Next, the constraint matrix is accepted where one row corresponds a single constraint as was demonstrated in Table 7.8. The fourth parameter is a vector of constraint directions referring to the `directionConstraints` column of the `lineupDF` data frame. The fifth parameter represents the "right-hand side" of the constraint direction meaning the right-hand side of the direction symbols. Finally, the `all.bin = TRUE` parameter dictates that the optimal solution should only have binary variables. This is because the use case represents binary player selections but in some optimization problems integers or even floating-point numbers could be the maximized or minimized optimum.

```
singleGame <- lp('max',
                 exampleSingleWk$game2022,
                 conMat,
                 lineupDF$directionConstraints,
                 lineupDF$lineupNeed,
                 all.bin = TRUE)
```

If one calls the object `singleGame` in the R console, the result is either "success" or "failure." For this single game a linear combination of constraints was a "success," and the maximized point value is printed to the console as 173.8511. The actual solution to the optimization captured as a vector of binary values where one corresponds to a player that was selected for the lineup and 0 is a non-selection. The code below accesses the binary vector `solution` first. The second line embeds this vector to the left of the comma so it can be used for row indexing. Again `which` is employed to create a Boolean evaluation of the `solution` vector. In these single simulated point outcomes for all players, the nine best selections to maximize points while adhering to constraints are shown in Table 7.11.

Table 7.11 The optimal lineup given the point totals for the simulated game 2022 among the 10,000.

Player	Position	Salary	Game2022
Evans, Mike	WR	6100	18.64
Watson, Deshaun	QB	7600	28.42
Cook, Dalvin	RB	8800	26.50
Godwin, Chris	WR	6000	20.58
Goedert, Dallas	TE	3600	10.22
Ozigbo, Devine	RB	4000	23.96
Lamb, CeeDee	WR	5300	19.22
Aiyuk, Brandon	WR	6700	19.63
Atlanta	DST	1900	6.62

```
singleGame$solution
exampleSingleWk[which(singleGame$solution == 1),]
```

In Table 7.11, representing a roster lineup for projected points in a single simulation, the constraints are upheld as follows:

- One defensive special teams group is selected—**Atlanta**
- One quarter back is selected—**Deshaun Watson**
- Up to three running backs are selected—**Devine Ozigbo, Dalvin Cook**
- One tight end is selected—**Dallas Goedert**
- Up to four wide receivers are selected—**Mike Evans, Chris Godwin, CeeDee Lamb, Brandon Aiyuk**
- The total lineup is equal to nine players—**the number of rows in the lineup is 9**
- The total salary amount is less than or equal to 50,000—**the salary sum equals 50,000**

The benefit of this analysis is not a single projected game. Any single game outcome that has been projected could be flawed. Instead, the optimization can be run 10,000 times and the most numerous selected players may be a good indication of a consistently successful lineup. The following code will run a loop from 1 to 10,000 iterating through the `i` variable and rerun the `lp` optimization for each loop. Each optimization requires a single `entireLeaguePlay` vector of points. This is selected dynamically by creating an indexing object `idx`. For example, when `i` is "2022," the `idx` object is concatenated with `paste0` to be `game2022`. This string is used in conjunction with `which` applied to the column names to create a Boolean outcome similar to previous code. The result is a dynamic single column data frame of points from the `rnorm` function that corresponds to a single observation for each of the players. It is dynamic because the vector of points will iterate from 1 to 10,000 programmatically. Next, with each pass of the loop, the single game outcomes are made to be dummy variables with `model.matrix`. As before, this information is row bound with `rbind` to the player count and salary information. In the following loop, the right-hand table of linear directions refers to the existing `lineupDF` columns because these are not changed. Each of the solutions is similar to the previous single game example. Therefore, each loop iteration solution consisting of binary selection is used to index within the `gameOutcomes` data frame. An additional column is appended called `oneLeaguePlay` which records the game identifier using the `idx` object. The final optimal lineup data frame is recorded within the list `optimalLineups`. Since the loop will rerun 10,000 times, the list of lineup solutions will have 10,000 elements.

```
optimalLineups <- list()
for(i in 1:nGames){
    idx <- paste0('game',i)
    print(idx)
    # Single project points across the entire league
    entireLeaguePlay <- gameOutcomes[,which(names(gameOutcomes)
==idx), with=F] # Entire league plays
    # Constraint Matrix
    conMat <- rbind(t(model.matrix(~ position + 0,gameOutcomes)),
                rep(1, nrow(gameOutcomes)),
```

```
                    gameOutcomes$DK.salary)
# Optimization
result <- lp('max',
             entireLeaguePlay,
             conMat,
             lineupDF$directionConstraints,
             lineupDF$lineupNeed,
             all.bin = TRUE) # all vars are binary
# Get the lineup solutions
results <- gameOutcomes[which(result$solution == 1),]
results$oneLeaguePlay <- idx
optimalLineups[[idx]] <- data.frame(name = results$Name,
                                    position =
results$position,
                                    lineup = idx)
}
```

This code will take some time to finish considering there are 10,000 optimizations to calculate. Luckily, the loop contains a `print` command referring to the `idx` object so the user knows the R session has not frozen and progress is being made. The 10,000 individual data frames can be flattened with `rbindlist` making analysis more straighforward.

```
allSolutions <- rbindlist(optimalLineups)
```

Once flattened, a simple analysis is to tally the most frequent players by position. A two-way tally can be obtained with `table` accepting two vectors. Here the count of the `position` and `name` columns are tabulated. The resulting object is a "table" class and can be changed to a data frame using `as.data.frame.matrix`. Using `grep` with the pattern "Baker" in the `colnames` of the data frame results in a column index 130. The is evaluated in the third code line to the right of the comma. The result is a small vector showing Baker Mayfield was selected as the optimal QB 301 times out of the possible 10,000 simulated scenarios. A quick way to identify the most optimal player by position is to apply the `max.col` function while indexing columns. Table 7.12 is the result of this function call showing the most numerous player position selections among all 10,000 scenarios. Keep in mind

Table 7.12 The most selected players among 10,000 simulated point optimizations.

	Atlanta	Allen, Josh	Kamara, Alvin	Kelce, Travis	Hill, Tyreek
DST	2236	0	0	0	0
QB	0	2399	0	0	0
RB	0	0	4571	0	0
TE	0	0	0	2628	0
WR	0	0	0	0	3412

this ignores the salary cap and does not account for the nine player lineup requirements, merely this shows the optimal single players.

```
playerTally <- table(allSolutions$position,
                     allSolutions$name)
topSelection <- as.data.frame.matrix(playerTally)
topSelection[,grep('Baker', colnames(topSelection))]
topSelection[,max.col(topSelection)]
```

Rather than reviewing single players, the top *N* players by position can be visualized. To obtain a "tidy" player position data object, the `%>%` can be employed to forward `allSolutions` to `group_by` and `count` as shown below. This will create a triplet matrix where the first column is `position`, the second `name`, and a third column `n` representing the count of the original `name` column.

```
playerTally <- allSolutions %>% group_by(position) %>%
count(name)
```

To construct a static plot, the triplet `playerTally` can be passed to the `ggplot` function. Within the function `filter` is applied there the position column equals `QB`. Next the aesthetics are declared so that the *x*-axis refers to the `name` column and *y*-axis refers to `n`. The *x*-axis declaration is nested inside `reorder` with `-n` to enforce the bar plot is ordered in a descending order. Dropping the minus sign will reverse the order to be ascending. The next layer, `geom_col`, adds columns referring to the previous `n` column. This differs from `geom_bar` which calculates the proportion of a value to determine the bar area. In contrast, `geom_col` accepts a vector of values. The last two layers adjust the aesthetics and rotate the *x*-axis text labels. Figure 7.2 is the resulting bar chart showing Josh Allen as the most frequent QB selection followed by Deshaun Watson.

```
ggplot(filter(playerTally, position == 'QB'),
       aes(x = reorder(name, -n), y = n)) +
  geom_col() + theme_hc() +
    theme(axis.text.x = element_text(angle = 90, vjust = 0.5,
hjust=1))
```

Since this plot can be cluttered and hard to interpret, a dynamic plot can aid the audience by providing a tooltip when the mouse cursor hovers above a bar. Using `echarts4r`, the following code will reconstruct a similar bar plot with the benefit of tool tips. First, `subset` the `topSelection` data frame to a specific position. This object retains positions as `rownames` attributes. In this example, the `DST` type is retained but can be adjusted for other positions. The result of the subsection is then transposed using `t`. In an effort to declutter the visual, another `subset` is applied to the transposed data to remove players or defensive units that were never selected, so the value must be `>0`. This performed within the `as.data.frame` function to change the object class from table to data frame. Then a new column is appended on the left side called `team` using the row attributes. Informationally this is duplicative but is needed because the `e_charts` function needs to

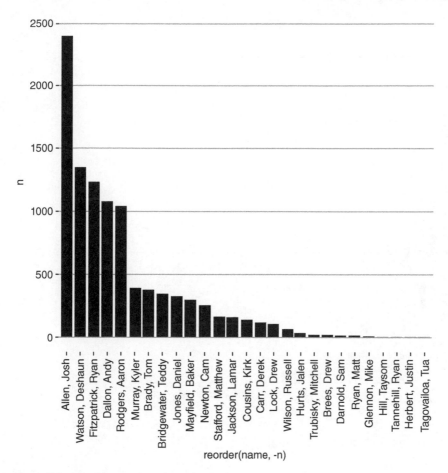

Figure 7.2 The QB selection frequency chart.

refer to a vector not an object attribute. Finally, the entire data frame is indexed according to the `order` function with the `DST` column and parameter `decreasing = TRUE`.

```
onlyDST <- t(subset(topSelection, rownames(topSelection)==
'DST'))
onlyDST <- as.data.frame(subset(onlyDST, onlyDST[,1]>0))
onlyDST$team <- rownames(onlyDST)
onlyDST <- onlyDST[order(onlyDST$DST, decreasing = T),]
```

The resulting `onlyDST` data frame is passed to `e_charts` to instantiate a blank visual. The x-axis is declared here as `team`. Similar to other tidyverse packages, there is no need to encase a column name with quotes. The bars are added with `e_bar` referring to the `DST` column. The next four layers improve the user experience of the visual by including

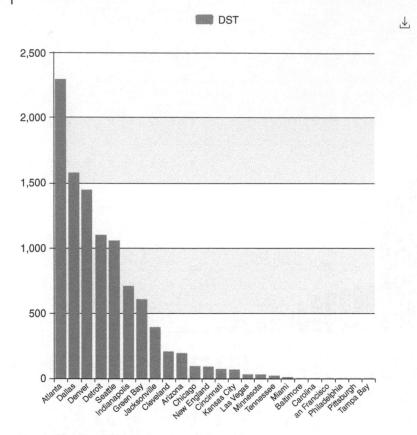

Figure 7.3 The DST bar chart from 'echarts4r'.

a tooltip, the ability for the plot to be saved as a static PNG file, rotating the axis labels, and applying a premade theme. The resulting dynamic plot has been saved a static image in Figure 7.3.

```
onlyDST %>%
e_charts(team) %>%
  e_bar(DST) %>%
  e_tooltip(trigger = "item") %>%
  e_toolbox_feature(feature = "saveAsImage") %>%
  e_x_axis(axisLabel = list(interval = 0, rotate = 45)) %>%
e_theme("gray")
```

Another way to visual frequently chosen optimized players is with a 'facet_grid'. The code below will select the top five values by position from the original tidy triple made previously. First a variable with value '5' is created call 'topN'. Next, this triplet is grouped using 'group_by' according to the 'position' variable. This is forwarded again to the 'top_n' function referring to the integer variable. Now the triplet is reduced from 186 positions to the top 5 for each of the 5 positions resulting in only 25 rows in the 'topPlayerSelections' object.

```
topN <- 5
topPlayerSelections <- playerTally %>% group_by(position) %>%
top_n(topN)
```

The reduced data set is passed to `ggplot` with the previous aesthetics in `aes`. The column declaration and theme layers are the same as before. However, the additional title layer is added with `ggtitle`. Additionally, the last layer will construct multiple bar charts in a grid. The `facet_grid` layer requires the dividing column name so that a bar chart is made for each factor level. In this case, a level corresponds to a position. The additional parameter allows the axis values to float rather than be explicitly aligned. This is needed because the frequency counts vary greatly between positions. Technically this parameter is optional and dependent on the data. Figure 7.4 demonstrates the application of `facet_grid` on the top-N data.

```
ggplot(topPlayerSelections, aes(x = reorder(name, -n), y = n)) +
  geom_col() +
  theme_hc() +
  theme(axis.text.x = element_text(angle = 90, vjust = 0.5,
hjust=1)) +
  ggtitle(paste('Top', topN,'Selections by Position')) +
  facet_grid(~position, scales = 'free')
```

The tabulated data can be joined to the `lineups` data for review to actuals since this is a historical look back. The `left_join` has the `playerTally` as the left table and columns two through six of `lineups` as the right side. The key column is case sensitive so the

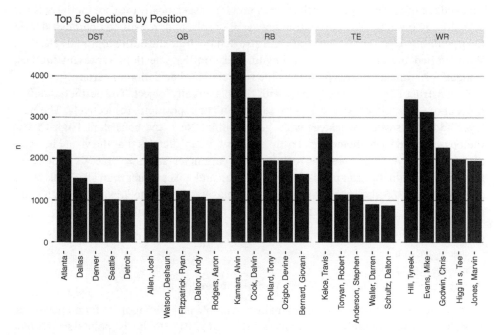

Figure 7.4 The facets bar charts by position.

Table 7.13 The joined optimal lineup tally and point information.

Position	Name	N	Points	Sd_pts	DK.points	DK.salary
DST	Cincinnati	65	4.56	1.06	2	2300
DST	Cleveland	209	5.96	1.85	6	3700
DST	Dallas	1539	5.8	1.93	10	2400
DST	Denver	1399	5.66	1l85	3	2300

declaration needs to be explicit as `by = c('name' = 'Name')`. Examining a portion of the join in Table 7.13 demonstrates that the `position`, `name`, and `n` (tally of optimal selection) have been joined with the projected `points`, `sd_pts`, and actual Draft Kings results in `DK.points`.

```
playerTally <- left_join(playerTally, lineups[,2:6],
by = c('name' = 'Name'))
playerTally[7:10,]
```

In this use case, the projected point standard deviation is a measure of uncertainty or risk. This is because the standard deviation impacts the width of the `rnorm` distribution. The standard deviation within the normal distribution represents the total range of possibilities for a player's earned points. With larger standard deviations, there is a greater number of point outcomes, wider kernel density plots. However, merely having a large point standard deviation does not necessarily mean the optimal lineup selects a particular player in most cases. Overall, there is a positive correlation between standard deviation and the number of optimal selections, but it is not specifically the case for the optimal selection by position. The correlation between `sd_pts` and `n` will be demonstrated in the upcoming scatter plot but the plot will also demonstrate the outlier optimal selection. With limited resources to choose a lineup, these outlier selections represent the best tradeoff for optimal reward (points) by the risk (standard deviation uncertainty).

To construct Figure 7.5 use `ggplot` with the `playerTally` object. The aesthetics define the x and y axes and color as columns `sd_pts`, `n`, and `position`, respectively. The next layer adds the scatter plot layer with `geom_point`. Next, the consistent High Charts theme is applied with `theme_hc`. Lastly the `facet_wrap` dictates that the visual is recreated for each level in the `position` column. The parameter `scales = "free"` is optional so that each individual scatter plot is free to float the x and y axes rather than all visuals being aligned. Figure 7.5 shows that outlier optimal players, where the `n` value is high compared to the `sd_pts` value, exist particularly for the non-DST positions.

```
ggplot(playerTally, aes(x = sd_pts, y = n, color = position)) +
  geom_point() +
  theme_hc() +
  facet_wrap(~position, scales = 'free')
```

The code below utilizes `rbokeh` to make a dynamic plot with tooltips for all positions. First, instantiate a `figure` and then forward that with `%>%` to the `ly_points` scatter plot layer. There are multiple parameters in this layer. First the column names for the x and y

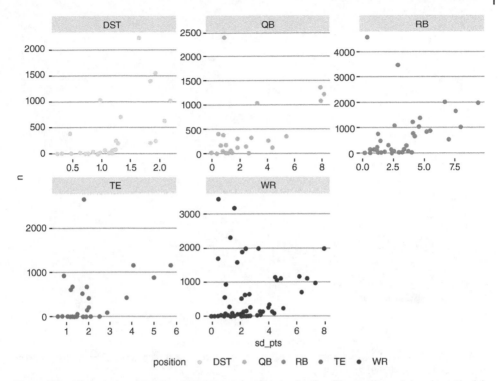

Figure 7.5 The relationship of uncertainty and optimal selection. The outlier points where the 'n' value yet the standard deviation is low represent possible optimal selections.

axes are input. Next, the data frame is passed in. The next two are merely aesthetics changing the point shape and the corresponding color according to the levels in the `position` column. The last parameter makes the visual more useful than a static plot. The `hover` parameter requires a list of column names when a user's mouse hovers over a point. Figure 7.6 is a static image of the JavaScript plot. If this plot is still too cluttered, the code after the visual construction creates a single `position` data object which can be input as the `data` parameter in the preceding code.

```
figure() %>%
  ly_points(sd_pts,
            n,
            data = playerTally,
            color = position,
            glyph = position,
            hover = list(position, name, n, points, sd_pts,
DK.salary))
# Single position alternative
riskReward <- playerTally %>% filter(position == 'TE')
```

Another way to explore the simulation results is by identifying the efficient players. One measure of efficiency could be the number of projected points divided by the salary cost.

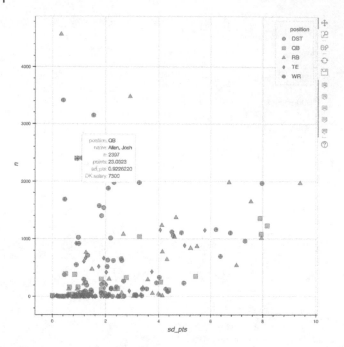

Figure 7.6 The HTML-based scatter plot between risk and reward by position. The outlier quarter back Josh Allen is shown as a tooltip.

Taken to an extreme, a player could be projected to have 0 points, and a salary of 9600 or more. This player would have a point per dollar value of 0 (0/9600). On the other end of the spectrum, a player's projection could 20 points with an accompanying salary of 3000. This player's points per dollar score would be 0.0066 (20/3000). Since salaries are in thousands the code below performs this operation and multiplies the result by 1000, though the multiplication is not technically needed. A new column `ptsPerDollar` is appended on the left side of the assignment operator using basic mathematical operations.

```
playerTally$ptsPerDollar <- (playerTally$points / player
Tally$DK.salary)*1000
```

Once an efficiency measure has been calculated, a preference selection can be made. In finance the capital asset pricing visual identifies an efficient frontier between risk and reward in a scatter plot. Similarly, this use case can also be understood in a three-dimensional market of risk, possibility and reward. The risk or uncertainty is captured in the `sd_pts` column. The possibility for an outcome is held within `n` and the reward is an efficient point acquisition demonstrated in the `ptsPerDollar` column. The `rPref` library helps identify a preference within a market using the `pSel` function. The code below employs `group_by` within the preference selection function so the selection so the selections are made for each `position`. Next, the preferences are declared. As a three-dimensional market problem, the optimal player has a `low` `sd_pts` uncertainty value, while retaining a `high` `n` possibility value and a `high` reward for point acquisition as `ptsPerDollar`. Each of these declarations is used within the following `psel` code and a portion of

Table 7.14 The preference selected QBs balancing risk, possibility, and reward.

Position	Name	N	Points	Sd_pts	DK.points	DK.salary	ptsPerDollar
QB	Allen, Josh	2397	23.03	0.92	35.30	7300	3.31
QB	Brady, Tom	382	21.00	0.84	32.92	6800	3.08
QB	Murray, Kyler	393	22.54	0.49	16.38	7500	3.00
QB	Ryan, Matt	13	18.86	0.001	22.90	5800	3.25
QB	Stafford, Matthew	165	18.33	0.96	0.68	5600	3.27

the results is displayed in Table 7.14. With the benefit of hindsight and known actuals in 'DK.points', it is clear that Josh Allen is the optimal QB. However, even without using the actual results, the optimization identified him as a top roster spot given the high 'n', low 'sd_pts', and high 'ptsPerDollar'. As a market, this player appears to be a good value for the salary given the high possibility he is optimal and the low uncertainty in projections. This contrasts with Kyler Murray who has a slightly more expensive salary, fewer projected points though smaller uncertainty. The tradeoff in risk and reward favors Josh Allen which was recognized in the optimization as 'n' and identified as a preferred selection in the code.

```
playerSelections <- psel(group_by(playerTally, position),
                         low(sd_pts) * high(n) *
high(ptsPerDollar))
as.data.frame(subset(playerSelections,
                     playerSelections$position=='QB'))
```

Perhaps a simpler approach is to only use 'psel' with 'low' for 'sd_pts' as a proxy for risk and 'high' for the projected points as the reward shown below. This resembles a more classic risk and reward tradeoff but widens the number of identifies player selections while not accounting for the optimization outcomes. Still if one has the ability to select multiple lineups perhaps this wider player selection data is best.

```
playerSelections2 <- psel(group_by(playerTally, position),
                          low(sd_pts) * high(points))
```

Regardless of which 'psel' object is used another single optimization can help identify the single best lineup from the efficient frontier players. Of course, there are many assumptions along the way along with opportunities for improvement. However, the results are sound and show significant advantage to choosing a single lineup. Since the entire population of players is now limited to the efficient players in 'playerSelections', the constraint matrix needs to be reconstructed. The 'model.matrix' data parameter needs to be updated along with the 'rep' function and, finally, the salary column too.

```
conMat <- rbind(t(model.matrix(~ position + 0,playerSelections)),
                rep(1, nrow(playerSelections)),
                playerSelections$DK.salary)
```

Table 7.15 The optimal lineup according to the optimization analysis for week 16 of the 2020 season.

Position	Name	Points	DK.points	DK.salary
DST	Atlanta	5.59	5	1900
QB	Allen, Josh	23.0	35.3	7300
RB	Gaskin, Myles	14.1	33.9	5300
RB	Kamara, Alvin	20.5	59.2	7900
TE	Goedert, Dallas	9.95	6.8	360
WR	Cooper, Amari	16.0	19.1	5700
WR	Evans, Mike	16.7	43.1	6100
WR	Hill, Tyreek	21.9	10.5	9000
WR	Jeffery, Alshon	9.89	3.2	3200

Now another optimization is run with `lp` using the same direction and right-hand side table as before.

```
result <- lp('max',
             playerSelections$points,
             conMat,
             lineupDF$directionConstraints,
             lineupDF$lineupNeed,
             all.bin = TRUE)
```

Using code from before `which` is applied to the `solution` element of the optimization object. The resulting optimal lineup according to 10,000 simulated games is shared in Table 7.15. Additionally, the total projected `points` are ~138 but in actuality the results were even better, summing `DK.points` to more than 200 points.

```
optimal <- playerSelections[which(result$solution == 1),]
sum(optimal$points)
sum(optimal$DK.points)
```

Extend the Methods Employed

Obtain more sources to improve the standard deviation, improve imputationAccount for injuriesUsing fuzzy match for the player points and salaries joinImproved point projections with confidence intervals using ml algorithm. Then run rnorm to obtain the possible outcomesId the outlier playerFind the outlier player lineup that results in a minimum threshold of 140 pointsAdjust constraint matrix to get two sets of lineups with another rbind

Exercises

1) What is an optimization problem?

2) Why is `lp` a linear program or linear optimization? Can you provide an example of a linear optimization use case?

3) Rerun the analysis with a changed pointing schema based on another fantasy league's rules found online or simply document changing some parameters. Does this change the optimal lineups and player identified?

4) Rerun the analysis with the default point schema for week 10 within the 2020 season. Build a visual for the outlier players by position with `facet_wrap`.

5) In the preceding analysis, identify the preferred selection players using `psel` and identify an optimal lineup.

8

Exploratory Data Analysis

Searching Data for Opponent Insights

Objectives

- Download basic sports data
- Apply various functions to understand summary, tabular and statistical information of the data
- Build bar, timeline event, and line charts to explore patterns in the data
- Construct a Markov Chain to understand the next most likely event in an effort to more fully understand characteristics of the overall scenario represented in the data

R Libraries

```
ggplot2
ggthemes
pbapply
data.table
lubridate
dplyr
gridExtra
markovchain
RCurl
```

R Functions

```
library
<-
getURL
read.csv
```

Sports Analytics in Practice with R, First Edition. Ted Kwartler.
© 2022 John Wiley & Sons Ltd. Published 2022 by John Wiley & Sons Ltd.

```
summary
head
grepl
as.data.frame
table
aggregate
left_join
names
/
ggplot
aes
reorder
geom_col
theme_hc
ggtitle
grep
unique
t
subset
|
period_to_seconds
ms
geom_point
geom_vline
%in%
!
left_join
mdy
group_by
mutate
cumsum
summarise
max
geom_line
geom_text
theme
geom_smooth
prop.table
round
sample
unlist
markovchainFit
attributes
```

Sports Context

This chapter purposefully explores the data without a specific outcome. The methods employed meander by design and do not follow the SEMMA workflow illustrated elsewhere in the book. The code presented is meant to use basic data techniques to help a human make strategy decisions. In some analytical paradigms, a coaching strategy decision represents "human over the loop" decision(s) because the data only accounts for *measured* aspects of the game rather than accounting for qualitative or unmeasured aspects such as "being in the zone" such as externalities like a player having interpersonal off-court issues. Many analytical minded professionals have discounted non-measured variables like having a "hot hand" in basketball stating "the hot hand is a massive and widespread cognitive illusion."[1] All analytical measures are limited to observable and worthwhile variables for which one has access. Even the naysayers would admit that additional variables of value may improve game planning. For example, it is likely not feasible to measure each player's individual marital happiness or alcohol consumption when scouting an opposing team. Yet these non-measured humanistic aspects may be helpful in planning for an upcoming match. Thus, as with many complex business decisions, a data-driven coaching strategy may give an incomplete understanding in the moment. The result of this gap is that a coach or team leader must make instinctive decisions where data is supplemental. In the end, the game outcome and accountability lie with the leadership staff. Surely no professional coach has been able to save their job after losing seasons simply by stating "the data made me do it."

This chapter is the result of 6–8 h of exploratory work in an effort to mimic the undertakings of a business analyst assigned to support a coaching staff. In practice, the visuals and data-based conclusions would be integrated into a coaching or leader's thinking on the game, conference, or league yet would not dictate the decision-making.

This chapter focuses on Women's Collegiate Division I Soccer (Futbol, Football, or Footy to non-US readers) data. The commonplace exploratory techniques are covered though not robustly because the book covers some data exploration in most chapters. Additionally, this chapter does not cover spatial analysis which is often performed with soccer nor does it cover advanced statistics and modeled outcomes like expected goals. These caveats exist because spatial data is reviewed in the baseball chapter and advanced statistics including spatial coordinate data are not readily available for the Women's game. Collectively these analyses are covered in the book not within a Women's soccer context. However, the code does create interesting visuals supporting a data narrative to be given to a decision maker and presents an advanced exploratory technique to understand the probabilistic nature of game states.

This analysis mimics a realistic situation in data analysis. Often there is a database with multiple tables. If the database is relational, there is a unique key or identifier so observations can be combined. While database queries and joins are outside the scope of this chapter, the code below employs multiple tables with differing fidelity and summarizations or statistics of the data. For example, a single team plays multiple opposing teams throughout a season. Additionally, a single team consists of a roster with individual player

---

1 Kahneman, D. (2011). *Thinking, fast and slow.* Farrar, Straus and Giroux.

performance. Thus, a game summary is the summation of a team's effort and outcome while individual player information may be aggregated not to a single game but to a seasonal level. As a data practitioner care must be taken for proper data joins, temporal matching such as season-to-season data or within a season and grain including individual player statistics compared to team level aggregate data.

Specifically, this chapter focuses on women's soccer teams within "Mid-American Conference" or MAC for the 2019 season. The MAC consists of 12 collegiate teams[2] shown in Table 8.1. The exploration focuses on the University of Akron Women's team. It is being performed from the perspective of an analyst supporting either an opposing team leadership seeking to understand Akron's 2019 weaknesses and style in the hopes it will indicate the upcoming season's play. On the other hand, an Akron coach could use this information in the offseason to identify and improve areas of opportunity. As previously mentioned, more complete data would yield additional insights and as a data exploration chapter the reader is encouraged to update and add to the data while also expanding on the code examples.

According to the US National Collegiate Athletic Association, NCAA, the following basic soccer data is defined below.[3] This chapter focuses on these basics in an effort aid learning for EDA while other chapters are devoted to predictive and explanatory methods.

- Shot—A shot is an attempt that is taken with the intent of scoring and is directed toward the goal.
- Assists—An assist is awarded for a pass leading directly to a goal.
- Goal—An offensive player who either kicks or heads the ball into the goal is awarded a goal.

Table 8.1 The MAC teams within this chapter's data.

	University	Abbreviation in data
1	University of Akron	AKR
2	Bowling Green State University	BGSU
3	Ball State University	BSU
4	Buffalo	BUF
5	Central Michigan University	CMU
6	Eastern Michigan University	EMU
7	Kent State University	KSU
8	Miami University (OH)	MIA
9	Northern Illinois University	NIU
10	Ohio University	OHIO
11	University of Toledo	TOL
12	Western Michigan University	WMU

---

2 NCAA. (n.d.). *Mid-American conference*. Mid-American Conference. https://getsomemaction.com.

3 IHSAA Boys Soccer. (2012). SOCCER STATISTICS GUIDE. Indianapolis.

While this analysis focuses on goals and shots as fundamental statistics, a number of additional engineered variables are capable of being calculated. These statistics should be part of a complete EDA project and can be applied to players and teams. While the code does not focus on these statistics as particularly insightful, they are demonstrated in a basic manner. More of this chapter's text is devoted to visuals and a more nuanced exploratory analysis method called a transition matrix.

- Goals per game—Total goals divided by total games played.
- Assists per game—Total assists divided by total games played.
- Points per game—Total points per game divided by total games played. *Where one point is awarded for an assist and two points are awarded for a goal.* This is not to be confused with goals per game which is a raw count of the goals scored.

Finally, the data was sourced directly from the official MAC website. At the time of writing, the following link contains the data tables. As a result, the reader is encouraged to update for subsequent seasons as well as identify additional and likely more complete statistics for exploration yielding additional insights.

- https://getsomemaction.com/stats.aspx?path=wsoc&year=2019

Technical Context

Overall, this chapter uses basic R programming for summary statistics and visualizations.

However, a more advanced exploratory data analysis technique explores the transition probabilities of in game play action. An effect of a soccer game is a series of events captured in play types throughout an individual game. For instance, a shot may be deflected out of bounds by a defending player which results in a corner kick. The corner kick may be well placed and result in another shot or a goal. These chains of events and their corresponding probabilities can be constructed programmatically, then understood qualitatively to help understand opponent propensities such as offensive aggression or lack thereof. For example, constructing a transition matrix of an opponent may indicate the opponent is more successful than others are turning a corner kick into a goal which could impact on-field decision-making.

In fact, these transition states of nature are used in many disciplines such as stock trading.[4] While this chapter is merely reviewing the transition probability matrix as part of exploratory analysis, it is an artifact of Markov Chain analysis. A Markov Chain is a statistical technique based on transitions from one state to another according to a given set of probabilistic rules.[5]

A Markov Chain analysis reviews segments of state changes in a series. The changes can be of varying lengths and a "fit" Markov Chain can predict future states from the

---

4 Amunategui, M. (2016, September 16). *Predict stock-market behavior using Markov chains and R*. Data Exploration & Machine Learning, Hands-on. https://amunategui.github.io/markov-chains/index.html.

5 Carrera Arias, F. J. (2018, August 30). *Markov chain analysis in R*. DataCamp Community. https://www.datacamp.com/community/tutorials/markov-chain-analysis-r.

historical probabilities of changes between states. Consider the following small example similar to the upcoming data. Here, a small set of play sequences are artificially constructed in the `seq` object which is similar to the package documentation's example but modified to be soccer related.[6]

```
seq <- c('SHOT', 'CORNER', 'GOAL', 'SHOT', 'GOAL',
         'SHOT', 'SHOT', 'CORNER','CORNER', 'SHOT',
         'GOAL', 'CORNER', 'SHOT', 'SHOT', 'SHOT',
         'SHOT', 'CORNER','GOAL', 'GOAL')
```

If one tabulates the first-order transitional states, for example, from "SHOT" to "CORNER" or other states like "SHOT" to "GOAL," one can then extract probabilities. The transitial sequence matrix is easily obtained from this data with `createSequenceMatrix`. This creates an "n" by "n" square matrix where the number of rows equals the number of columns. To interpret the matrix shown in Table 8.2, one should focus on the row first. The row represents the first action in the sequence while the column represents the secondary result. For example in the preceding `seq` vector "CORNER" followed by "CORNER" appeared once. Thus, the intersection of row-CORNER and column-CORNER has one as a value. Similarly, scanning the sequence one would find two occurrences of a "CORNER" next transitioning to a "SHOT." In contrast, a "SHOT" turns into a "CORNER" three times so the row-SHOT and column-CORNER intersection has a different value than the transposition CORNER to SHOT.

Our focus is first-order transitions given the lack of data, play action chains that may be interrupted in the data compared to reality, and the fast moving pace of soccer in general makes a second or tertiary Markov Chain investigation difficult and likely uninformative. This may not be the case with complete or different data such as men's or professional play types or in other disciplines.

Further, since the data presented in this chapter is incomplete, a Markov Chain model is not very useful though the underlying play probability transitions may be. There are two reasons for the limited use of a proper Markov Chain model. On one hand, an in-game model is of limited use in a high paced game such as soccer, where decisions are made instinctively among these top athletes. Additionally, the data is incomplete where some plays like a simple midfield pass up field are not recorded plus results in the limited data have states of transition with 0.00 probability of occurring so the model

Table 8.2 The sequence matrix demonstrating sequence action tallies.

	CORNER	GOAL	SHOT
CORNER	1	2	2
GOAL	1	1	2
SHOT	3	2	4

---

6 Spedicato, G. A. (2017, August 16). Crash Introduction to markovchain R package. Nexr.com. http://cran.nexr.com/web/packages/markovchain/vignettes/markovchainCrashIntro.pdf.

would never accept a transition to one of these states. For example, later in this chapter one team's transition matrix of plays have no headers resulting in a foul. While it may not be likely that a header would result in a foul it must certainly happen from time to time in normal game play, just not in this data set. For these two reasons, a Markov Chain may be insufficient for team leadership. In contrast, the transition matrix can help in overall game strategy, one where a coach may remind the team from the sideline that once an opponent has committed a foul, they are very likely to take a shot for their next play perhaps out of strategy or frustration at the foul among other transition probabilities. Another positive of a play action analysis is that it will not take many games to accumulate some understanding of play transitions, and these can be updated as the season progresses. This chapter uses season ending data, but the transition matrix would remain effective with partial data though get more trustworthy as the season progressed. Of course, there would be high variability and even a cold-start problem in game one and earlier in the season.

Code- Exploratory Data Analysis

To begin, the following URLS are available in the public book repository. Each URL string corresponds to hosted CSV files making, `gameXwalk`, `macPlays`, and `roster` representing game summary information, intragame actions by time and individual team player seasonal summary statistics, respectively. If the intent is to explore a different team, the `roster` URL will need to be updated to another team roster in the repository.

```
gameXwalk <- 'https://raw.githubusercontent.com/kwartler/
Practical_Sports_Analytics/main/C8_Data/MACgameInfo_table.csv'
macPlays <- 'https://raw.githubusercontent.com/kwartler/
Practical_Sports_Analytics/main/C8_Data/macPlays_2019_2.csv'
roster <- 'https://raw.githubusercontent.com/kwartler/
Practical_Sports_Analytics/main/C8_Data/teamRosters/AKR_
seasonRoster_summaryStats.csv'
```

Next, using the URL string objects applies `getURL` to download the individual files from the repository. The function employs `libcurl` inside the function to perform the request and retrieval of the data.

```
gameXwalk <- getURL(gameXwalk)
macPlays  <- getURL(macPlays)
roster    <- getURL(roster)
```

Finally, the `read.csv` function reads the downloaded file. In each of the preceding steps, the objects `gameXwalk`, `macPlays`, and `roster` are simply overwritten to avoid clutter within the r-session environment.

```
gameXwalk <- read.csv(text = gameXwalk)
macPlays  <- read.csv(text = macPlays)
roster    <- read.csv(text = roster)
```

In an effort to avoid coding duplication, a single string is captured as the `team` object. Here, the exploration is performed with the University of Akron which is shortened in the data to `AKR`. This string could be changed to any of the schools within the data repository. Specifically, the strings could be `BGSU`, `BSU`, `BUF`, `CMU`, `EMU`, `KSU`, `MIA`, `NIU`, `OHIO`, `TOL`, and `WMU`.

```
team <- 'AKR'
```

Obviously, R basic EDA functions. Some of the common ones include `summary` and `head`. The `summary` function can be applied to any object and in the case of data frames will provide column-wise information depending on the vector type. For example, if the column is numeric, the minimum, quartile, median, mean, maximum, and number of NA's is returned. In contrast, limited information is returned for character vectors while factor level information is tabulated along with an NA count. Another common function is `head` which defaults to printing the first six rows of a data frame. Here, these functions are applied to all three objects to get a basic understanding of the data frames. Keep in mind there are other useful common EDA functions like `names` and `dim` providing column names and row, column numbers, respectively.

```
summary(gameXwalk)
summary(macPlays)
summary(roster)
head(gameXwalk)
head(macPlays)
head(roster)
```

The next level basic statistics outlined by the NCAA include "goals per game," "assists per game," and "points per game" as defined previously. The `roster` data frame contains the required data to calculate this information at the player level. If one wants to explore these statistics at the team level, all rosters are needed from the book repository. Within `roster`, there is a `TEAM` entry representing the statistical summaries for the single school and the individual players. For now, the calculations are performed to understand the impactful players for the University of Akron 2019 team. The goal is to identify characteristics of individual players for a fictitious upcoming match.

The `gpg` goals per game data frame is constructed with `name` vector and a simple vectorized calculation dividing the `shot_stats.goals` vector by `games_played`. The original `games_played` and `shot_stats.goals` columns are retained for context in case a player only plays a single game yet scores which would inflate this statistic. Then, `head` is applied to the data frame to examine the first six rows of the two-column object. Within the `head` call the code is employing `order` with parameter `decreasing` equal to TRUE. This is to the left of the comma so that the rows are ordered by the new calculated statistic.

```
gpg <- data.frame(name = roster$name,
                  games = roster$games_played,
                  goal = roster$shot_stats.goals,
                  shots = roster$shot_stats.shots,
                  gpg = roster$shot_stats.goals/roster$games_
played) head(gpg[order(gpg$gpg, decreasing = T), ])
```

As noticed in the ordered six rows, the players Ashley Amato and Carly Pcholinksy played in 19 games with high goals per game statistic. A contextualizing statistic may be to review a player's shots on goal divided by overall shots. A shot "on goal" is one that is within the dimensions of the goal net, requiring a save by the goalie, or a defender. A shot that hits a goal crossbar or post without a defending team deflection or is wider or higher than the net is a shot that is *not* on goal. The code constructs a new column `onGoal-Rate` by dividing the column `shot_stats.shots_on_goal` by `shot_stats.shots`. This could be a measure of a player's propensity to shoot even without a clear line of sight, equating to offensive aggression or a player's poor shot placement when taking an otherwise good shot, where the kick is on goal but easily saved by the defense. Table 8.3 shows the results of this small data frame when the previous `head` and `order` code is reapplied. Table 8.3 may indicate that Bailee Bowers could be more aggressive when taking shots because her on goal rate is considerably higher than other goal per game leaders. If this is the case and it fits within overall team strategy, coaching may want to encourage her to take more shots. In contrast, Aislinn Meany took an astonishing 61 shots in the season. Her on goal rate was relatively good considering the number of shots overall but it may be the case that the coaching strategy should focus on getting this prolific shooter more "good looks." Of course, these statistics are without context, and care must be taken to incorporate insights into lineup or strategy changes.

```
gpg$onGoalRate <- roster$shot_stats.shots_on_goal /
  roster$shot_stats.shots
```

Calculating both assists per game and points per game is straightforward with the additional columns `shots_stats.assists` and `shot_stats.points`. In fact, the `roster` data set supports multiple additional engineered variables.

```
gpg$assistPerGame <- roster$shot_stats.assists / gpg$games
gpg$pointsPerGame <- roster$shot_stats.points / gpg$games
```

Any of the engineered statistics can be quickly visualized as a bar chart. The code below has some nuances worth noting. First, the `gpg` data frame is passed to `ggplot` containing a logical condition. Here, the `gpg$shots>0` Boolean result determines inclusion in the data received. One needs to ensure the logical check is to the left of the comma to ensure it is applied to rows. Next, the aesthetics are set up with `aes`. The default behavior of `ggplot` is to accept factors as presented, here

Table 8.3 The outlier on goal rate and shot statistics pertain to Bailee Bowers and Asilinn Meany, respectively.

Name	Games	Goal	Shots	Gpg	onGoalRate
Amato, Ashley	19	5	23	.263	.565
Pcholinky, Carly	19	5	29	.263	.586
Worthy, Sydney	20	3	16	.15	.562
Bowers, Bailee	20	2	7	.1	.714
Meany, Aislinn	20	2	61	.1	.426
Brown, Abigail	18	1	5	.05	.4

alphabetically. This makes the visual difficult to interpret so `reorder` is applied. The *x*-axis represents player names but reordered by the shots value. The minus sign means the reorder is done in a decreasing manner. Of course, the *y*-axis is appropriately defined as the `shots` variable. Since this is a column chart, the `geom_col` layer is added next. The last three layers, `theme_hc`, `theme`, and `ggtitle`, improve aesthetics with predefined palates, rotated *x*-axis labels, and a simple title, respectively. Figure 8.1 is the example bar chart for total shots but the code can easily be adjusted for other statistics in the data object, just remember to change the logical condition in the first layer.

```
ggplot(gpg[gpg$shots>0,],
          aes(x = reorder(name,-shots), y = shots)) +
  geom_col() +
  theme_hc() +
  theme(axis.text.x = element_text(angle = 90,
                                      vjust = 0.5, hjust=1)) +
  ggtitle(paste(team, 'shots'))
```

Moving to the `macPlays` object, the granularity of the data is different. Rather than player level season level information, this data has data within a single game. There are over 10,000 rows representing individual plays among the games. The caveat as mentioned earlier is that the data is not complete due to the differences among recording methods school to school. Some data cleaning was applied to unify team abbreviations

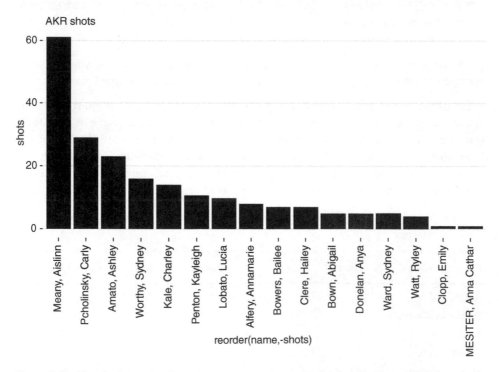

Figure 8.1 Akron's players by shots demonstrate a power distribution similar to Zipf's law.

and other data aspects, but it is likely additional cleaning steps could further improve the pending insights.

As seen when calling `head` on `macPlays`, the column `action` specifies the type of play undertaken. Two additional vectors of TRUE or FALSE are reconstructed below. The function `grepl` is a pattern matching function that has a logical return, hence the "L" ending the `grep`. The first input is the string to be searched. In this example, the string "SHOT" and "GOAL" are anchored using `\\b`. This is the regular expression representation of a backspace. This additional anchoring in the string means the pattern "GOALIE" will not be counted while the fixed "GOAL" will be. There are other packages that perform common string tasks like `stringi` and `stringr` including finding fixed string patterns. The `grepl` function is a base R operation. The second parameter is the search vector and the last is an optional Boolean parameter whether capitalization should impact the search operation. This code engineers two new columns `shot` and `goal` for later use.

```
macPlays$shot <- grepl('\\bSHOT\\b', macPlays$action, ignore.
case = T)
macPlays$goal <- grepl('\\bGOAL\\b', macPlays$action, ignore.
case = T)
```

Using the newly created `shot` column, an aggregation is applied to the `macPlays` data. Since R interprets Boolean TRUE and FALSE as 1 and 0 the aggregation can `sum` the TRUE values. Here, the formula is `shot` by `team` followed by the data set and finally the function to be applied. The resulting `shotsInData` object is a small data frame summing the total shots for a team in the data, for example, AKR having 175 shots in the season and BGSU with 290.

```
shotsInData <- aggregate(shot~team, macPlays, sum)
```

Next, a tabulation of all included teams in the data set is performed using the `gameX-walk` data frame. First, the `c` combine function concatenates the `homTeamID` and `awayTeamID` vector into a single longer vector. This is tabulated with `table`. Finally, the object is converted to a data frame and saved as the `totalGames` object. The result is the total number of team occurrences identified within the `gameXwalk` data frame such as Youngstown State University (YSU) appearing three times.

```
totalGames <- as.data.frame(table(c(gameXwalk$homeTeamID,
                                     gameXwalk$awayTeamID)))
```

Bringing these two summary tables together is performed with a `left_join`. The left hand table is the `shotsInData` followed by `totalGames`. The key column is defined as `team` in the left table and `Var1` which is a default name when `table` is applied then converted to a data frame. As a left join, the non-MAC teams are dropped when constructing the `shotsGames` object.

```
shotsGames <- left_join(shotsInData,
                        totalGames,
                        by = c('team' = 'Var1'))
```

The following code simply names the third column as "games." The `names` function is on the left of the assignment operator with square brackets and an index of `3` so that only that position is declared with the assignment operation.

```
names(shotsGames)[3] <- 'games'
```

Next, a simple calculation at the team level contrasts the previous individual player example. The `shotsPerGame` variable is left side declared by dividing the `shots` column by the `games` column.

```
shotsGames$shotsPerGame <- shotsGames$shot / shotsGames$games
```

This team level information is similarly visualized in Figure 8.2. The following code accepts the tabulated and joined data `shotsGames`. The *x*-axis is a reordered `shotsPerGame` column in a decreasing order while *y*-axis is simply the `shotsPerGame`. Then, `geom_col` declares the type of visual followed by simple aesthetics of `theme_hc` and `ggtitle`. This type of view may contextualize teams that have offensive prowess and when reviewed along with conference standings may inform coaching staff for the minimum viable number of shots needed to be a top tier team. Of course, this assumes all shots are of equal probability for success. Since quality of shot matters, one could reconstruct this visual with additional `grepl` engineering on the play `text` column to identify shots that were wide versus `"BLOCKED"` similar to the previous shots on goal description. Still this basic visual likely has correlation to team standings and knowledgeable coaching staffs can incorporate this into their upcoming strategy thinking.

```
ggplot(shotsGames,
       aes(x = reorder(team,-shotsPerGame), y = shotsPerGame)) +
  geom_col() +
  theme_hc() +
  ggtitle('Avg Shots Per Game')
```

To this point, the exploration was basic. However, the play data represents novel viewpoints that can be investigated effectively through visualization. First, let's create an `idx` index object using `grep`. Unlike `grepl` which returns the logical result if a character pattern was found one or more times, dropping the "L" will return the index position if the pattern was identified one or more times. Here, `grep` accepts the `team` object representing the string "AKR." The second parameter is the search space, the vector `team`. This indexing object of row positions is next used to subset the `macPlays` data frame into single team object, `oneTeam`.

```
idx <- grep(team, macPlays$team)
oneTeam <- macPlays[idx, ]
```

If interested, one can examine the unique game identifiers with `unique` to demonstrate the retained games from among all MAC plays. Additionally, if one wants to explore the distribution play types, a simple `table` call applied to the `action` column suffices. Rather than change the data class and manipulate the data further, a double transposition `t` nesting another `t` prints the data vertically for quick yet effective exploration.

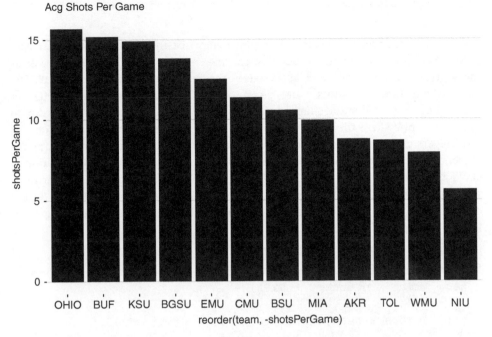

Acg Shots Per Game

Figure 8.2 The team average shots per game throughout the season.

```
unique(oneTeam$gID)
t(t(table(oneTeam$action)))
```

Since it is likely the case that a goal resulted from a shot, the single team plays are further subset to only these specific play actions. Using `subset` applied to the `oneTeam` data frame, the second parameter is a logical condition. However, the logical condition actually represents to checks and an OR operator. First, the logical condition checks if the `action` column is equal to `GOAL`. Then, a "pipe" operator, a vertical line usually above a keyboard's enter key, represents an OR logical operator. After the pipe operator, the second logical check is employed returning TRUE if the `action` is equal to `SHOT`.

```
oneTeamShots <- subset(oneTeam,
                oneTeam$action=='GOAL' |
                oneTeam$action=='SHOT')
```

The time for each game is a continuous number of seconds. However, the data is provided with minutes colon and seconds. Thus, a conversion is needed. The new column is left constructed with called `gameSeconds` by employing `lubridate`'s `period_to_seconds` function. The `period_to_seconds` function needs a numeric time object so another function, `ms`, is first applied to the original `clock` vector. The `ms` function stands for minutes and seconds. It will attempt to parse string characters into a `lubridate` object class called "period." In the end, a string such as "03:10" is parsed to a period as "3M 10S," then parsed again to 190 total seconds (60 * 3 + 10) as the new numeric `gameSeconds` vector.

```
oneTeamShots$gameSeconds <- period_to_seconds(ms(oneTeamShots$
clock))
```

Next, let's construct a "Cleveland Dot Plot" to more easily interrogate the 700+ data points. Set up the plot using `ggplot` with `oneTeamShots`. Declare the *x*-axis as the continuous `gameSeconds` and *y*-axis as the factor unique identifiers `gID`. The next layer instantiates points using `geom_point` where the action-type SHOT or GOAL dictates the color and shape. A vertical line at the half-time mark is added with `geom_vline` where the *x*-intercept is 2700 s. Lastly, the `theme_hc` and `ggtitle` layers change the layout while adding a dynamic chart title using the `team` object. The resulting visual is illustrated in Figure 8.3. As a coach the distribution of shots and goals appears to be relatively dispersed throughout the game supporting a well-conditioned squad. However, this may not be the case for other teams in the data. Perhaps teams get off to an aggressive start while others have to make up ground later in the game.

```
ggplot(oneTeamShots, aes(x = gameSeconds, y = gID)) +
  geom_point(aes(color=action, shape = action),size = 3.5) +
  geom_vline(xintercept = 2700) +
  theme_hc() +
  ggtitle(paste(team, 'shots & goals over time'))
```

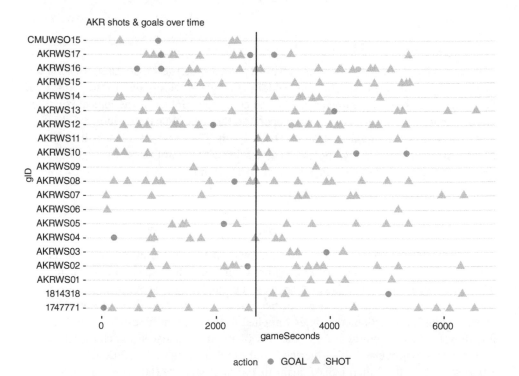

Figure 8.3 The Cleveland dot plot showing Akron's dispersal of shots and goals for each game.

As a coach you may also want to know how opponents have fared against Akron's team. While the `gameXwalk` has this data, it can be obtained using the original `macPlays` data and the `oneTeam` objects. First, identify the `unique` game ID's where Akron played. This is the second parameter to the `%in%` value matching operation. The first is the vector of all `macPlays$gID`. The result is a vector of positions where the unique IDs are matched between the two vectors. This is to the left of the comma to select appropriate rows from the entire `macPlays` data frame. In the end, the `oppTeam` object captures only soccer players where Akron was involved.

```
oppTeam <- macPlays[macPlays$gID %in% unique(oneTeam$gID),]
```

At this point, the `oppTeam` data consists of all soccer players including Akron and the opponents. One method to remove the Akron plays is with another `grepl` where the pattern is `AKR` applied to the `team` column. Next, the `oppIdx` Boolean vector is switched with the negation operator, `!`. This will switch TRUE to FALSE and vice versa. The effect is that any time "AKR" was found with `grepl`, the Boolean vector is now changed to FALSE. This vector is placed inside square brackets to the left of the comma to perform the subset of the `oppTeam` data frame.

```
oppIdx <- grepl('AKR', oppTeam$team)
oppTeam <- oppTeam[!oppIdx,]
```

For clarity, Akron's opposing team shots are ignored in favor of only `GOAL` actions. This will reduce visual clutter for the audience. Here, `subset` is applied with a single logical condition where the `action` column is equal to `GOAL`. Next, the conversion from string to periods to count of seconds is reapplied as was described previously.

```
oppTeamShots <- subset(oppTeam, oppTeam$action=='GOAL')
oppTeamShots$gameSeconds <- period_to_seconds(ms(oppTeamShots$
clock))
```

Figure 8.4 is a reconstruction of the Cleveland dot plot but only for Akron's opposing teams and only for goals. Although there may be data integrity issues as mentioned multiple times in this chapter, this visual clearly shows that Akron's defensive vigilance wanes in the second half of the game. It appears as though opposing teams have more success scoring after half time. If the following `ggplot` code is unclear at this point, review the code chunk for the previous figure for a more detailed explanation.

```
ggplot(oppTeamShots, aes(x = gameSeconds, y = gID)) +
  geom_point(aes(color=action, shape = action), size = 3.5) +
  geom_vline(xintercept = 2700) +
  theme_hc() +
  ggtitle('Opponent Goals over time')
```

Another perspective may help understand teams that are consistent throughout the season for various statistics. It may be the case that some teams will start the season successfully then lose momentum as the season grinds on. One method to explore this is by reviewing a cumulative sum and plotting the cumulative sum as a line chart. Of course, this data represents a complete season, but the upcoming visual could be useful later

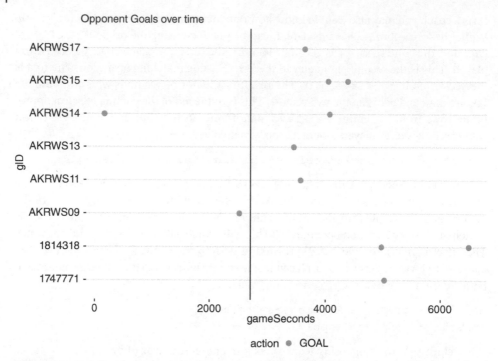

Figure 8.4 The Cleveland dot plot demonstrating opposing team Goal success in the second half of matches.

within a season to understand a team's endurance or consistency. A coach could review the upcoming chart noting a slowing rate of shots or other statistic and make strategy choices to improve in subsequent games, perhaps by focusing late season practices on these diminishing efforts. The drawback of the upcoming chart is that it is not useful early in a season until significant games have been played.

First, using `gameXwalk` join the game date to the play action data. The left side table that is retained completely is the `macPlays` data frame. On the right, only the `gID` and `date` columns are retained because that is the only variable needed. As a result, the key vector is the `gID`. The `date` column is then parsed from a character string to a date class using `lubridate`"s `mdy` since the format is month, day, and year in the original string.

```
macPlays <- left_join(macPlays, gameXwalk[,1:2], by = "gID")
macPlays$date <- mdy(macPlays$date)
```

To ensure the data is presented correctly, the `macPlays` data frame is ordered within square brackets similarly described previously.

```
macPlays <- macPlays[order(macPlays$date), ]
```

Next, using `dplyr`"s `group_by` function, each team's cumulative shots are calculated. Since the data was ordered in the preceding code, only `team` is used in the `group_by` function. While `date` may be redundant considering the previous `order`, it may avoid incorrect outcomes in similar data sets. The `%>%` pipe forwarding

Table 8.4 The cumulative results within a single game that was engineered in code.

gID	Shot	csumShots
1739048	FALSE	0
1739048	FALSE	0
1739048	FALSE	0
1739048	FALSE	0
1739048	TRUE	1
1739048	FALSE	1
1739048	TRUE	2
1739048	FALSE	2
1739048	TRUE	3
1739048	FALSE	3

operator will forward the grouped data to `mutate` to construct a new variable. The new variable name is `csumShots` and it is derived with the base-R `cumsum` function applied to the `shot` column. As an exploratory analysis, the visual can be constructed with other statistics extracted from the `action` column. Finally, the `macPlays` data class is changed to the base-R data frame with an empty `as.data.frame` call. Table 8.4 is an abridged result demonstrating the new column and cumulative effect of calling the first 10 rows where TRUE is accumulated over play action time.

```
macPlays <- macPlays %>% group_by(team) %>%
  mutate(csumShots = cumsum(shot)) %>% as.data.frame()
head(macPlays[,c(1,12,15)],10)
```

To make the visualization more informative, another variable is calculated. Here, `maxByTeam` is constructed by `group_by` according to team. Then, each team's section of the data is subjected to `summarize`. This function is purposefully built to accept grouped data in `dplyr` and return fewer rows according to some additional logic or calculation. In this case, the column `maxShots` is created simply by extracting the maximum value for each team's previously engineered `csumShots`. Another variable is created after the comma applying similar logic to the `date` column. The goal here is to extract the *x–y* coordinates for each team's cumulative shots for use in the visualization.

```
maxByTeam <- macPlays %>% group_by(team) %>%
  summarise(maxShots = max(csumShots, na.rm = T),
            maxDate = max(date, na.rm = T))
```

Let's start by creating the first few layers of the plot in an object called `p1`. Using `ggplot` pass in the `macPlays` data where aesthetics are defined as `x=date`, `y= csumshots`, and color and group are defined by `team`. Next add the `geom_line` layer along with a standardized `theme_hc`.

```
pl <- ggplot(macPlays, aes(x=date,
                           y=csumShots,
                           colour=team,
                           group=team)) +
  geom_line(size=1, alpha=0.25) +
  theme_few()
```

Now the `pl` plot has a `geom_point` and `geom_text` layers added. The difference is that the `data` parameter is set to the maximum data frame, `maxByTeam`. The *x–y* coordinates are similar to the previous line layer but instead will be a single point placed at the end of each team's line or in the case of `geom_text` the team's abbreviated name. Lastly, another `theme` is added to remove the default legend. The result of this code is illustrated in Figure 8.5. In Figure 8.5, one can observe a higher cluster of teams while there is also a middling cluster and a lone lagging team according to this statistic. Reviewing league success will demonstrate a correlation to the shot rate observed in the chart and final league standings. Keep in mind this is not known until the end of the season and the real benefit of reviewing a chart like this among other statistics is to note which aspects of the game a roster may be less enduring which may need additional practice attention or alternatively to exploit against.

```
pl +
  geom_point(data = maxByTeam, aes(x     = maxDate,
                                   y     = maxShots,
                                   group = team,
                                   color = team), size = 2) +
```

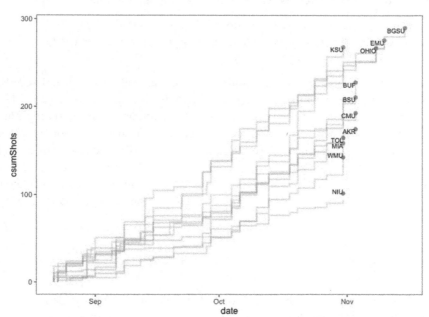

Figure 8.5 The cumulative shots over the season where the slope indicates higher shot rates over the season.

```
geom_text(data = maxByTeam, aes(x    = maxDate,
                                 y    = maxShots,
                                 group = team,
                                 label=team),
           color = 'black', hjust = "inward", vjust = "inward",
size = 3) +
theme(legend.position = "none")
```

An alternative to this visual is to construct the lines with a smoothing function. Instead of `geom_line` which will have explicit values, the layer below utilizes `geom_smooth`. The rest of the layers remain unchanged. For some audiences, this smoothed look is more informative than the step-up version considering the data is looking for an accelerating or decelerating statistical trend. According to `ggplot2` documentation, `geom_smoth` aids the audience to represent patterns when there is overplotting or visual clutter.

```
ggplot(macPlays, aes(x=date,
                      y=csumShots,
                      colour=team,
                      group=team)) +
  geom_smooth(method = "loess") +
  theme_few() +
  geom_text(data = maxByTeam, aes(x    = maxDate,
                                   y    = maxShots,
                                   group = team,
                                   label = team),
             color = 'black',
             hjust = "inward",
             vjust = 1.5,
             size = 3,
             fontface = "bold") +
  theme(legend.position = "none")
```

To aid in understanding for a black and white publication, Figure 8.6 is a modified version of the preceding smoothed line chart. Three teams are highlighted for comparison while the other team lines are made grey and dashed. In Figure 8.6, Ohio University remained a top shooting team throughout the 2019 season. The University of Akron was less prolific but consistent given their almost straight line. Interestingly, a top achieving team, Bowling Green State University started shooting at a much higher rate later in the season as evidenced by the increasing slope moving the line from the middle of the pack to the upper cluster of teams.

Constructing Akron's transition probability matrix for play actions starts with first understanding the team's overall actions in the data. Using the `oneTeam` data frame for Akron's subsection of the `macPlays` data, a tabulation can be performed for the action types. Here, `table` is nested inside `prop.table` to create proportions of the whole rather than raw value counts. Table 8.5 shows the 12 play types along with proportion and raw count.

```
prop.table(table(oneTeam$action))
```

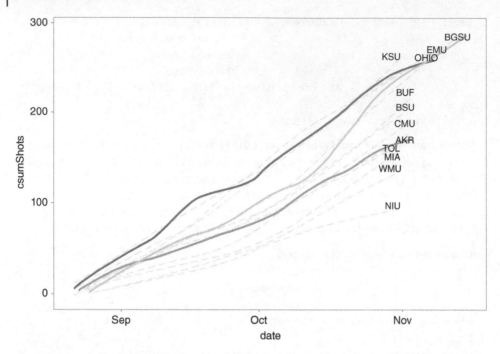

Figure 8.6 The adjusted smoothed line chart showing cumulative shots throughout the season.

Table 8.5 The tabulation and proportion of Akron's play type.

Play Action	Proportion	Count
CORNER	0.100	72
FOR	0.015	11
FOUL	0.271	195
GOAL	0.026	19
GOALIE	0.038	28
GOLMSG	0.005	4
HDR	0.016	12
OFFSIDE	0.077	56
PENSHOT	0.004	3
SHOT	0.243	175
SUB	0.176	127
YC	0.022	16

As was done previously, the `ms` minute and second parsing function is nested within `period_to_seconds` to sum the play action time log to total seconds since the game start. Some of the teams in the data have NA listed for the time stamp. If that is the case, a warning is printed to the console noting that some periods failed to parse. To account for this one can use `complete.cases` on the constructed `gameSeconds` vector to the left of the comma to create a Boolean which drops the unparsed observations. To avoid the parsing warning, the parameter `quiet` can be set to FALSE but this is not conservative data manipulation! If all timestamps parsed, the second line will have no effect.

```
oneTeam$gameSeconds <- period_to_seconds(ms(oneTeam$clock,
                                            quiet = F))
oneTeam <- oneTeam[complete.cases(oneTeam$gameSeconds),]
```

There are timestamps within games that last longer than 90 min and these are dropped from the data set because the "stoppage" time likely changes normal transitional game-play. Teams playing in this added time may be more aggressive taking wild shots since time is running out. Since the timestamps were converted to seconds, a logical condition is created where seconds less than or equal to 5400 (90 min × 60 s) are retained. This limits the transitional states to the more normal gameplay.

```
oneTeam <- oneTeam[oneTeam$gameSeconds<5400, ]
```

In case one game had a significant shortage of logged plays or the opposite where a game constitutes an outlier in terms of number of plays a simple `table` call on the `gID` column will be needed. The goal is to identify any problematic games though the Akron data has a consistent number of actions per game. There are two games which have twice as many logged plays as others but overall, the number of plays is consistent among the rest. As a practitioner, one can remove the outlier games (both low or high), reduce their impact by capturing only a subsection of each, or simply leave them intact within the data. Although there are two games with outliers in the Akron data, the games will remain without adjustment. The analysis could easily be rerun to understand the impact and the point of the code is to inform the practitioner.

```
table(oneTeam$gID)
```

Although there is a chapter devoted to simulation regarding fantasy football lineups, a similar approach can be undertaken with EDA. In some cases, using synthesized data is acceptable and moreover is a growing research field within machine learning. Here, the data is relatively small yet play states as "chains" of events can be reconstructed because they do not start only at the beginning of a game. The loop to construct synthetic data ignores play transitions interrupted by quarters and half time for simplicity's sake and improve learning but could be improved by incorporating additional logic.

The loop to construct synthetic play chains will run 10,000 times where `i` is iterated upon. First, a simple `print` call will alert the practitioner the loop's progress. Next, a single game is randomly sample as the `randoGame` object. This line employs `sample` to select one of the `unique` game identifiers. Next the single game is subset from the data and retained as `oneGame`. This is performed using a logical operator to the left of the comma in square brackets where the game identifier is equal to `randoGame`. Next, play series quantity is randomly created. As a design choice, the length of a chain is 5–10 actions and a single number from the `5:10` vector is sampled. This helps emulate the fact that some plays may only be a few actions while others may be multiple in series. Although the transition matrix is not a model, this can be thought of as a tuning parameter of the synthetic data construction. Next, the stream of events should begin at random times so another sample is applied. Here, the starting row is determined from the first row to the total number of rows in the single game data *minus* the `seriesQty` integer. This ensures the chain will be complete and that the loop will not cause an error. In the end, a single chain of 5–10 play actions is selected starting from anywhere within the game plays. For example, five plays could be selected starting on row 11 for a specific game (play actions 11, 12, 13, 14, 15 from game A) and the next time through the loop, seven plays could be selected starting on the second line from a different game (play actions 2, 3, 4, 5, 6, 7, 8 from game B). Finally, to construct a single series, `oneGame` is subset using indexing and these sampled integers. Rows are selected to the left of the comma starting with `seriesSt` and extending to the sum of `seriesSt` and `seriesQty`. To the right of the comma only the sixth column, play `action` is retained in this manner. Although only a single vector, it is technically a data frame, so the data is passed to `unlist`. The last line merely appends the vectors of varying length actions into a list. In the end, the loop creates a list of 10,000 vectors with different lengths. Each vector represents a chain of play actions from actual game data.

```
randoSeries <- list()
for (i in 1:10000) {
  print(i)
  randoGame <- sample(unique(team$gID),1)
  oneGame <- team[team$gID==randoGame,]
  seriesQty <- sample(5:10, 1)
  seriesSt <- sample(1:(nrow(oneGame) - seriesQty), 1)
  seriesSection <- oneGame[seriesSt:(seriesSt + seriesQty), 6]
  randoSeries[[i]] <- unlist(seriesSection)
}
```

The library `markovchain` has a convenient function that will build the chain while also embedding a transition matrix. The `markovchainFit` function can accept a list, character vector, or square matrices as mentioned in the technical explanation section. The loop's list can be passed without further manipulation.

```
mcFit <- markovchainFit(data = randoSeries)
```

The resulting object is an "S4" type which means accessing elements is slightly different than traditional "S3" R-objects. These class types are at the discretion of the package author and are said to be optimized and more correct programming though less popular. Any new R programmer can get confused as to how to access elements of an S4 object but is shown here as an example and also to extract the transition matrix rather than to merely extract the matrix immediately.

One can call `class` on the Markov Chain fit like any other R object. The result is a simple list. Next, the `attributes` function helps to identify the S4 elements or "slots."

```
class(mcFit)
attributes(mcFit)
```

The interesting aspects of the `mcFit` object is the `estimate` slot. Now one can reapply `class` and `attributes` so dig a level deeper in the object investigation. The `estimate` slot is of class `markovchain` which is not informative. Next, the `attributes` of this subelement includes noteworthy information.

```
class(mcFit$estimate)
attributes(mcFit$estimate)
```

The `attributes` call prints the following elements to the console:

- `states`—a vector of the unique states found among all 10,000 vectors.
- `byrow`—Boolean if the Transition matrix was constructed by rows.
- `transitionMatrix`—the matrix of probabilities among all combinations of states.
- `name`—the type of chain constructed; not particularly applicable in this context but for those interested readers, either MLE employing a "Laplacian Smoother," bootstrap, or Bayesian inference. The default MLE was used in the code example.
- `class`—the object class which is a custom "markovchain" type for the markovchain package.

After reviewing the attributes print out, it is clear the single element needed is the `transitionMatrix`. Here is where selecting data within S4 objects can be different than S3 objects. For educational purposes, the `mcFit` object can have the `estimate` selected using a `$` sign similar to most complex and named R objects. However, the next level slot for data is accessed not with a `$` but with `@` within S4 object types. The first code line below accesses only the vector of unique states found in the data. R programmers may try to use `$` for both the first and second level elements as shown in the second code line, but this will yield an error, "$ operator not defined for this S4 class."

```
mcFit$estimate@states
mcFit$estimate$states
```

Thus, it is straightforward to obtain any data element once one realizes how to access a specific S4 slot. Here, the `@` is employed to select just the transition matrix and capture it as an object called `transitionMat`.

```
transitionMat <- mcFit$estimate@transitionMatrix
```

Table 8.6 is a rounded version of the transition matrix from the University of Akron's women's team with 2019 seasonal data. Keep in mind, the play chains were synthetically created so individual results may vary slightly.

To interpret the transition matrix, one starts with the first state represented in rows and then finds the corresponding column for the next play state. For example, a CORNER kick will result in another CORNER kick immediately as the next play with a 0.15 probability. In comparison, an OFFSIDE (row) will have 0.39 and 0.21 probabilities for a SUB (substitution) or FOUL, respectively, as the next play action. To make complete use of a transition matrix, a coach could have one created for an upcoming opponent noting the most likely next outcomes for their opponent in game. Additionally, reviewing all teams' transition matrices within the context of winning, top-tier teams may help a coaching staff in the off-season to focus on play states where top teams excel compared to others. For example, BGSU may have differing transitional states off of corner kicks compared to other teams.

Table 8.6 Akron's play transition state for the 2019 season.

	CORNER	FOR	FOUL	GOAL	GOALIE	OFFSIDE	PENSHOT	RC	SHOT	SUB	YC
CORNER	0.15	0.00	0.27	0.03	0.00	0.13	0.03	0.00	0.25	0.12	0.02
FOR	0.00	0.00	0.00	0.00	0.00	0.00	0.00	0.00	0.00	1.00	0.00
FOUL	0.05	0.04	0.26	0.02	0.00	0.11	0.00	0.00	0.08	0.38	0.05
GOAL	0.00	0.00	0.33	0.00	0.00	0.00	0.00	0.00	0.00	0.67	0.00
GOALIE	0.17	0.00	0.27	0.05	0.00	0.16	0.00	0.00	0.40	0.00	0.00
OFFSIDE	0.06	0.06	0.21	0.00	0.00	0.10	0.00	0.00	0.13	0.39	0.00
PENSHOT	0.00	0.00	0.00	0.00	0.00	0.00	0.00	0.00	0.00	1.00	0.00
RC	0.00	0.00	0.00	0.00	0.00	0.00	0.00	0.00	0.00	1.00	0.00
SHOT	0.09	0.00	0.20	0.03	0.00	0.05	0.00	0.00	0.25	0.36	0.02
SUB	0.04	0.02	0.17	0.00	0.00	0.05	0.00	0.00	0.12	0.60	0.01
YC	0.05	0.13	0.47	0.00	0.00	0.00	0.00	0.08	0.08	0.12	0.07

Exercises

1) Reconstruct the Cleveland Dot Plot with NIU, Northern Illinois University. Review the 2019 MAC Women's soccer standings. What does this chart say about NIU's style of play or contexualize about their opponents?

2) Compare the NIU, AKR, KSU, and BGSU Cleveland Dot Plots. Without knowing the final standings do these charts help you understand each squad's ability? Which team appears to be the best, middle, and one with the most opportunity for improvement? If you were AKR's coach and you received KSU's first 100 plays charted this way, what should be focused on? Should the AKR coach focus on Kent State's first half-defense or instructing the team to be more vigilant in the second half? Sharing only the first 100 rows mimics in season progress rather than complete data after the fact.

3) Create a cumulative sum chart based on team Corners. As a measure of overall offensive pressure not explicit shots, do top teams create more corner kicks? Are they consistent throughout the season?

4) Construct BGSU and NIU transition probability matrices. Reviewing the relationship between CORNER and GOAL play states which team turns a corner kick into a shot with higher probabilities? Which team kicks a CORNER and has a higher probability of a FOUL? Does this data support a coaching focus for NIU to improve in one area of the game to get parity with a top performing team?

Index

Sports Analytics in Practice with R, First Edition. Ted Kwartler.
© 2022 John Wiley & Sons Ltd. Published 2022 by John Wiley & Sons Ltd.